QUILT ON FIRE

BY THE SAME AUTHOR

FICTION

Tiny Sunbirds, Far Away

Where Women Are Kings

NON-FICTION

The Language of Kindness

The Courage to Care

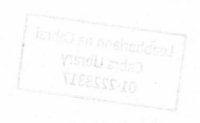

QUILT ON FIRE

The Messy Magic of Midlife

Christie Watson

Chatto & Windus
LONDON

1 3 5 7 9 10 8 6 4 2

Chatto & Windus, an imprint of Vintage, is part of the Penguin Random
House group of companies whose addresses can be found at
global.penguinrandomhouse.com

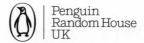

Penguin
Random House
UK

First published by Chatto & Windus in 2022

penguin.co.uk/vintage

A CIP catalogue record for this book is available from the British Library
HB ISBN 9781784744045
TPB ISBN 9781784744052

Typeset in 10/18 pt MillerText by Jouve UK, Milton Keynes

Printed and bound in Great Britain by Clays Ltd, Elcograf S.p.A.

The authorised representative in the EEA is Penguin Random House Ireland,
Morrison Chambers, 32 Nassau Street, Dublin D02 YH68

Penguin Random House is committed to a sustainable future for
our business, our readers and our planet. This book is made from
Forest Stewardship Council® certified paper.

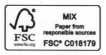

For my mum. And her mum. And her mum.

Contents

Author's Note

This book is based on real events. However, some names and details have been changed in order to protect identities. Joy, for example, is made of composite experiences. Alastair is an entirely fictionalised character.

1

The Desert in Utah: Mind

I am invisible. I finally got what I wanted. My brother and I spent much of our childhood arguing about superpowers: would it be better to be invisible or to be able to fly? As a child I often dreamt I was flying and would claim that nothing could beat that feeling of speed and freedom, the giddy whoosh of being in the night sky. 'Invisibility,' my brother would tell me, leaning in and whispering as if it were a secret, 'means you can spy on people. You can know *everything*.' Eventually we would both agree that to see without being seen would be the greatest of all powers.

Yet here I am, invisible, and I feel totally and utterly helpless.

I am sitting in the car outside Sainsbury's and people are walking past me without so much as a glance in my direction. I look straight at them with a swollen, crying face, and nobody looks back at me. I've never really been a crier. I can watch the saddest of films without shedding a tear. My nurse heart, I've often thought, is a bit hard and brittle around the edges. I can laugh a lot, be incredibly sarcastic, sometimes sardonic, and have developed the dark protective humour of my profession. Yet here I am, a blubbering, snot-crying wreck. I feel like running, too. Away from something I can't quite name. My leg muscles are tense, on high alert, as if they want to bolt. I remember my friend Joy, after her son was born, phoning me up in a panic. She told me she'd been putting the bins out when she looked down the lane and had suddenly wanted to run. Run away and never come back. She described the longing for freedom, to be herself once more, without carrying the weight of another life. 'I wanted to leg it. To run fast as my legs could carry me. I looked into the distance and every single bone in my body screamed at me to run.' I feel like that now: like packing it all in, running for the hills. I watch people walking past, resolutely oblivious to me, as I sit in the car staring out at them. In a full, busy car park, I feel very alone. And just *wrong* somehow. I feel like I'm floating outside my own skin, looking down at myself, but all I can see is a faint outline, a shell, emptied of organs, vacant. I can't articulate these feelings, not even to friends and family; I can't seem to relate to anyone, except perhaps Mrs Dalloway: 'She had a perpetual sense, as she watched the taxi cabs, of being out, far out to the sea and alone; she always had the feeling that it was very, very dangerous to live even one day.' Perhaps it is insomnia? For the first time in my life, I am not sleeping. I've been waking, routinely, every night at 3 a.m. foam-mouthed, shaking and sweating with anxiety, like a rabid dog.

Am I a terrible mother? Is the world ending? Did I turn the oven off? Did I pay the parking fine? Is my TV licence up to date? Will I go to prison? Who will take care of the children?

I worry about everything, but mostly about my teen children. They have been watching me suspiciously, recently, as if I am possessed. They move past me cautiously staring, a little confused, and when they ask, 'How was your day?' in bright, breezy voices, I tell them, good, great, *I'm fine*, and ask about theirs, but instead of sounding reassuring, my voice sounds artificial, saccharine.

I spend an entire weekend staring at the television screen. The only problem is that the television is turned off.

I search every morning for my keys, which I keep in the zipped part of my bag. They are never there when I first look. I scour the house, the kids' bedrooms, even the oven and fridge, where I do keep finding random things: my wallet, passport, a lipstick. Finally, when I check my bag again, they are there – suggesting they were there all along. 'I don't believe you,' I tell the keys. Even the keys look worried.

I get out of the car slowly and head into the shop. I always pick the trolley with the dodgy wheel, which is a bit of a metaphor for my love life, really. My trolley today, though, is worse than unmanageable, so I give up and grab a discarded basket.

I look at the rows and rows of food and my head spins. All I need to do is buy food to fill the almost entirely empty fridge and cupboards and make sure there are dinners. The basics. And yet it feels like a mammoth task. I don't care; it's as though I have no care left, it's been totally rinsed out of me. I'm empty of it, this woman's resource that is assumed unending. I have suffered compassion fatigue in my nursing career before, but this is something entirely different. Care fatigue? A woman walks past with a shopping list, checking things off as she goes, aggressively ticking. I can't plan. I walk down the aisles quickly, and chuck random items into the basket as if I'm doing Supermarket Sweep. Pasties, courgettes, Mini Cheddars, tinned sweetcorn. I am burning hot. My legs and feet stop working properly. I suddenly shuffle as if weighted down, through the aisles, and my eyes blur. I feel the cool coming out of the freezer section, and stop. People walk past, ignoring me still. I must be sick. Flashes and dots float inside my eyes. I open a glass door, the shelves behind it half empty of fish fingers, and lean in, and in, until I am able to half close the door. The air is cold on my back and I feel sweat drip down my spine, almost in relief. The icy blast on my body goosebumps me into calm, and I take a few deep breaths. My head settles and I come to a pause, half in a freezer, next to the fish fingers, frozen in all senses. I should feel humiliated. I often do. I'm standing in a freezer. Surely, I should be cold-water swimming, like everyone else seems to be, all those women who are doing life better? But instead of getting out of my fish finger freezer, I watch the other shoppers walk past, dare them to say something, anything. I lean into the cold. Still nobody looks at me. They aren't averting their eyes, embarrassed, or pretending to be on the phone; they simply carry on as if they can't see me. One man comes over to the freezer next to mine, opens it, takes out some breaded cod, then closes it, without a flicker of awareness that I am there.

It's as I stand here in this freezer, transparent, see-through, quite possibly mad, that I understand that I need to take urgent action. Michel Foucault said in *Madness and Civilization*, 'Madness, in its wild, untamable words, proclaims its own meaning; in its chimeras, it utters a secret truth.' I want to know my secret truth. But the only person who understands me is a chronically depressed – and arguably narcissistic and bourgeois – fictional Virginia Woolf character. I am unravelling in a spectacular fashion. I need help simply to function. And also, fuck invisibility, I still want to fly.

Luisa is an older woman, dressed brightly in cheerful summer colours. She has a wise face that is somewhere between kind and stern, a lived-in expression of someone who has seen, up close, humanity at its most mysterious and perhaps unimaginable. Hers is the face of an older nurse. 'We will fill out these forms at the start of each session. It's a good way for us to record your progress.' She nods to the pieces of paper she has left on the chair opposite her. I pick them up, tick boxes about how I'm feeling. I have no idea how I'm feeling. I skim down and scribble random answers anyway. I hand the forms back to her, and watch as she reads my answers, knowing they are all wrong.

There's a print of that famous Japanese woodcut, Hokusai's *The Great Wave*, on the magnolia wall. I turn to stare at it for a while, and imagine the crashing of water engulfing me, the relief. I imagine drowning. I can't afford therapy. But like many women, I *really* can't afford to be sick. 'Honestly, as a single parent I felt I didn't have the time to deal with dark thoughts,' a friend tells me after a major depressive episode. I look away from *The Great Wave*.

Searching for a therapist seems like it should be straightforward but I found it anything but. Therapy is an unregulated industry, which feels particularly dangerous. I have done my homework, asked around, and found Luisa, who is based in a clinic on the outskirts of north London.

'What brings you to me today?' She half-nods and half-smiles; carefully curated movements. It's a sunny day and dust particles float between us. The dust moves slowly, as though the air is sad. Sad air. I think of all the people who must have sat here, breathing out sad air, until it changed the atmosphere itself.

I have googled every possible mental health issue and

taken every quiz available on the internet, and discovered I apparently have the same personality type as Malala Yousafzai and Barack Obama, which only makes me feel utterly inadequate. I must have some sort of untreatable neurological disorder, or end-stage undiagnosed syphilis or Lyme disease or an incurable mould allergy that will mean I need to go and live in the desert in Utah.

I don't tell Luisa this. I do not mention neurosis. Instead, I talk about feeling unseen. I've never felt myself to be a particularly beautiful woman. Striking, possibly–in the right light–but not head-turningly stunning. Yet I always noticed the glances, the slightly too long stares, and the subtle–and not-so-subtle– flirting that made me *feel* seen by men, and by women. 'When I was younger, I imagined that I wouldn't miss being visible in our patriarchal society and its obsession with the young, the fetishisation of youth, and external, sexualised ideas of beauty. But now that I'm becoming invisible, and I have the ability to see without being seen, I realise that I was wrong. I mean, I know how strange I sound, but I feel totally not there. Like I'm creeping away from being real or something.'

Luisa doesn't ask about my anxiety, or my low mood, which I've ticked on the forms, or the self-diagnosed breakdown (I climbed into the fish finger freezer in Sainsbury's, I tell her. I *hard relate* to Mrs Dalloway).

She doesn't even frown. Poker faces are important for

therapists too, I realise, thinking about my twenty years as a nurse, my own poker face. Instead, she asks me about my age, and about my periods. I'm confused as to why she's even asking. 'It's as if I've got insects crawling all over my body,' I tell her, in a bid to prove that my psychological state is pathological and serious. 'I am totally disconnected to my sense of self, outside my body, outside my own reality. I fantasise about disappearing, running off to join an ashram, somewhere far away. I'm not right,' I tell her. I describe looking in the mirror and wondering who I am, or at least, where I have gone. 'I feel empty. And like something catastrophic is happening in my brain and my body.'

She doesn't say anything, but her careful listening, half-nodding, half-smiling propels me on. I describe the anxiety nights, the neurotic days, the feeling that I have no idea who I am any more, and I reiterate that everything is distorted. 'I'm worried I'm really sick,' I say, crying. All I seem to do is cry these days. 'And I'm not a crier.' There are strategically placed tissues next to my chair, I notice. 'I'm losing it. My body is falling apart. And my brain is mashed potato. I'm a writer. An academic. I can't read – all I do is watch reality TV. I need a working brain.'

She waits until I finish blowing my nose. 'This could all be hormones,' she says. 'I think you need to see your GP in the first instance. Of course we will carry on talking, if you think it would be helpful, but I do think it's wise to get your hormones checked too. Sounds like the kind of thing a lot of women experience at perimenopause.'

Perimenopause? The word is becoming more familiar, with a much-needed movement of women speaking out publicly and in the media about their experiences of both perimenopause and menopause. But at this point, I only recognise the term in a vague sense. A sing-song word, quite beautiful said out loud: *perimenopause.* But I've not really heard it as anything but passing conversation.

The word 'peri' comes from Greek *peri* (prep) and means 'around, about, enclosing'. I certainly feel enclosed, constricted, not held in a calm and reassuring way, but squeezed. But surely I'm nowhere around the time of menopause? I thought that happened mid- to late-fifties? Something to shelve and worry about later. And anyway, if this were a common thing experienced by women, wouldn't we be talking about it all the time? Surely lots of women don't all have colossal breakdowns, quietly, *invisibly...* I am surprised and sceptical about Luisa's advice. I can't believe that these enormous emotions I'm unable to contain are down to hormones. To getting older. In her TED Talk 'How to Live Passionately – No Matter Your Age', the novelist Isabel Allende said, 'For a vain female like myself, it's very hard to age in this culture. Inside I feel good, I feel charming, seductive, sexy. Nobody else sees that.' I also feel like

I'm disappearing, like I am vanishing. And I hate it. I am vain. But is this really about my simply getting older, and my vanity? A hormonal imbalance might be part of the story, of course, but there must be something far deeper going on. This tumult is too big, too uncontrolled, to be related to menopause.

The word 'menopause' was invented by French (male) doctors at the beginning of the nineteenth century. Some of them noted that peasant women had no complaints about the end of menses, while urban middle-class women had many troubling symptoms. I wonder why women had such different experiences. I have troubling symptoms. Yet I feel as if I do not know myself at all. I am urban, it is true, and, although I grew up very working class, could now for sure be considered middle class. My situation is more than troubling: it's debilitating. I am swimming in syrup. And surely troubling symptoms happen at the time of menopause, not a decade beforehand? I don't even *feel* menopausal. But what do I know about the menopause, really, other than what I imagine it to be?

I later discover that although menopause typically occurs at forty-nine to fifty-two years old, it can begin earlier. It varies from person to person, with 80 per cent of women having their last period between the ages of forty-four to fifty-eight. And it varies from country to country, too: the average age of a woman's last period in the UK is fifty-two, but in India it's forty-four. So it's nearly upon me, a turning point, a pause of re-evaluation, *the change*, but at forty-two I am surely not there yet. But then I find out that women who work nights – just as I did for many years as a nurse – can reach the menopause a full decade earlier. And experience the perimenopause even younger. Perimenopause, the before, is something for which I am totally and utterly unprepared. And when I try and find information about it there is no clear-cut advice; instead, there are tons of contradictory explanations and theories. The time leading up to the menopause, this perimenopausal state, according to the North American Menopause society, can last between four to eight years. But the NHS website tells me that one in ten women experience perimenopausal symptoms for up to twelve years. *Harvard Health* describes perimenopause as the 'rocky road to menopause', but I'd never really considered that it might make women feel totally unhinged. Let alone that it would happen to me. Surely, this madness can't be attributed to perimenopause, and surely it can't go on for *a dozen years*.

Luisa looks at me again, with pity. 'Middle age can be a really hard time.'

I feel my heart flip over.

A memory lands on my skin of a tiny baby I cared for who was born with his heart completely the wrong way around, a condition called, quite grandly, Transposition of the Great Arteries. He was entirely blue-grey, the colour of steel. I remember his recession, the way his chest folded in half with each breath, his sternum becoming a small pit, and I remember blowing bubbles above him, and one popping on his nose, the sound of him giggling.

These memories that haunt me should ground me, remind me how lucky I am. How insignificant my problems are. I tell Luisa how guilty I feel to be so self-obsessed.

'The forties can be a profound emotional adjustment for women,' Luisa tells me. As though she can read my mind. 'Then the change of life,' she says. 'Perhaps the biggest transformation of all.'

'Would you prefer bubblegum or olive oil?' Krisztina, a different sort of therapist, is stirring a pot full of hot wax with a wooden stick. I'm lying on a reclining bed, watching *Friends* on a wall-mounted TV to take my mind off the fact that I'm completely naked from the waist down. Krisztina – who is probably sick of *Friends* – pays no notice to my embarrassment. In *The Coming of Age*, Simone de Beauvoir wrote, 'until the moment of it is upon us, old age is something that only affects other people.' I am shocked at my sudden, changing body, and my response is this. The room smells of lavender and babywipes. There are small bins everywhere, a chair on which I have carefully folded my jeans on top of my knickers, and the walls are painted lilac. Next to me a trolley contains a few large pots that look like something you might cook rice in but contain hot wax in different colours, a cup filled with wooden sticks, like those small forks you get at traditional fish and chip shops, maybe tongue depressors, a few pairs of tweezers in antiseptic fluid, scissors both small and large (shears, almost, presumably for extreme circs) and a handheld mirror. Krisztina briefly studies my face, as if trying to imagine the type of person I am. 'Olive oil then,' she says. I am an olive oil person, it is true. 'Lift your legs to your bum and drop them to the sides.' She smothers my vulva with hot olive-green wax and waits. There is no smell of olive oil, but I'm hoping it is somehow gentle on my skin. Olive oil certainly sounds more natural than bubblegum. Though as both a nurse and a woman who has given birth, I understand that natural rarely means gentle.

'We are great believers in olive oil in my family,' I say, trying to distract myself or Krisztina or both of us. I am full of embarrassment at the horror of the situation, of my strange body, and begin to ramble away as if words can cover nakedness. 'We use olive oil on hair, nails, skin,' I say. 'We even eat it on toast instead of butter.'

Krisztina ignores me, focusing on my naked half. She loosens the now hardened wax with her long, acrylic fingernails, and then she rips. The pain is quite unexpected, breathtaking, but it's over in seconds.

I smile, dementedly. But inside I am crying. I hate myself, how vain I am, how trivial and superficial and *basic*. Yet still, at forty-two, now I am *middle-aged*, and after discovering that my pubic hair is going grey, I am freaking out. Grey! I imagined dealing with grey hair on my head would be bad enough but when I find a couple of grey wiry pubic hairs, I am shocked. I hadn't even considered this possibility. It had never crossed my naive mind. Possibly worse still I have hair growing out of my chin, a moustache that makes me think of Frida Kahlo and then wonder why I can't be more like her. Surely this can't all be attributed to the perimenopause? This transformation feels simultaneously huge and peripheral. I find white eyebrow hairs that seem to grow straight outwards. I embark on car journeys with a pair of tweezers in my back pocket, as the light in the rearview mirror always shows up random black hairs that sprout from my face and even neck. Sometimes people going past start walking more quickly. Particularly men, I notice. There's clearly something frightening about a woman in a parked car plucking hair from her chin. I frighten myself. I feel like Jeff Goldblum in *The Fly*, thick black hairs erupting from my face and body. Grey hairs from my vulva. My body-horror film.

Luisa may be the first to identify my perimenopause, but the physical changes have, I realise, been going on for months, this Kafka-esque metamorphosis: hair loss (head), hair gain (everywhere else). I suddenly gained weight, and now regularly experience joint pain, night sweats, blurred vision, dryness, hay fever, gum problems, skin rashes, heart palpitations, abdominal disturbances. My body feels as if it no longer belongs to me.

I have so many questions about being a woman in my forties. Does everyone get grey pubic hair? Is this the beginning of the end? Or the end of the beginning? How many other women like me are changing like this, all at once, from a butterfly into a caterpillar?

I'd like to run away and never show my face, or indeed my naked bottom half, but here in this instance it's too late to turn back. My entire lower half is burning with pain. I hear the thrum of my own blood throbbing, on a loop, like an underwater alarm. I try to focus on this and not the anxiety whooshing through me about men who want women to look like pre-pubescent girls, and how I'm now complicit in that. 'I think that will do,' I say, looking at my baldness. But Krisztina smiles and scoops more wax with a wooden spoon, then spins round and pulls my legs up, smothering every crevice. She then leans towards me, frowning. I always think that things can't get any worse. But they often do.

'Put your legs higher up by your ears,' Krisztina says. 'So I can do your crack.'

Krisztina does not smile. She looks bored. I wonder if she herself waxes, or if she's embraced feminism in a way that I clearly haven't. I wonder whether she noticed my grey pubic hairs. She taps the wax with her fingers, then clearly realising it's another few seconds away from ready, starts to tidy up. Having felt the location of her fingertips and the wax I have rising anxiety about the possibility that maybe I have haemorrhoids, and the resultant blood loss if she accidentally tears one. I visualise blood on the ceiling. I imagine Krisztina as Carrie in the Stephen King film, blood rolling down her face. But it's over in a heartbeat, and with no injury. I lower my legs slowly and carefully to the *Friends'* theme tune.

Krisztina hands me a mirror. I look at her work, the baldness of me, like a naked mole rat; and feel like I'm the worst feminist in the world. That my ageing body fills me with horror is an uncomfortable truth. But still, I keep going back to Luisa's words: *middle age can be a really hard time.*

Middle-aged women do not book themselves into a Soho waxing bar for a Full Hollywood. Middle-aged women go to garden centres and have Pampered Chef parties and perfunctory sex with their middle-aged husbands. They know how to make butternut squash soup, how to wear scarves, and they get up early to meditate or do water aerobics. Middle-aged women make wreaths at Christmas and are on the PTA and watch *Strictly Come Dancing*. They use more than one setting on both the oven and the washing machine, and take multivitamins and have a skincare routine. Middle-aged women are well-behaved, mature beacons of society, and they understand stain removal and chop onions really well. Many of my friends, like me, are single, and regardless, we are all messy and complicated and behaving in many ways as we always have done since our teen years, maybe even a notch wilder. We are a bit frazzled, and often full of drama, sometimes debauchery. Is this middle-aged?

It's 2 a.m. and my friends and I are in a pub in Edinburgh shaking a vibrator machine that promises 'mini vibrators for six pounds each'. We are too drunk to understand that it is simply a gimmick and are disappointed that the machine does not release the goods. Emma high-kicks the machine; she's been doing kickboxing classes. Still nothing. False advertising! We complain to the management and are given sticky sweet shots of God-knows-what as compensation. Everything becomes even hazier after that and there are only flashes of memory. I open an emergency back door and two of my single friends are kissing random strangers, pressed against a wall. Emma has wandered off and returned in a new outfit, having swapped bras and tops with a stranger for no clear reason; Joy has joined the band and is playing the bagpipes (badly); Teniola is vomiting into an industrial bin. Samira is doing some sort of Highland dance on a flimsy table. Emma is back, doing her own dance move that belongs only in a strip bar. Large groups of people watch us, curiously. Some join in and laugh at our antics, others move away as if our loud exuberance is infectious. An old woman claps. We sing and shout and laugh and take the piss out of each other, and ourselves. Later, there is a terrible club: techno music and wasted teens. And we try and get a tattoo parlour to open, to adorn us with thistle tattoos on our ankles. Even later, there's another club, and some serious flirting with a group of men. One of the men joins us.

We wake bleary-eyed – in our apartment that looks like a Tracey Emin art installation from decades ago: empty bottles of cheap white wine and whisky, cigarette packets, half-smoked cigarettes, a pair of discarded Spanx, a traffic cone – to the screams of Emma, who cannot open her eyes. She has somehow used the wrong glue for her eyelash extensions. Panicking, I check my ankles, then breathe. No thistle. The random man is walking around topless, six pack on show, commenting that we are all a lot wilder than his friends, all in their thirties. He picks up a laminated itinerary that we had carefully prepared for the trip: *Arthur's Seat, Edinburgh Castle, Scottish National Portrait Gallery, Blair Street Underground Vaults* and starts to laugh. 'This is more what I imagined women your age would be like,' he says.

2

Year of the Dragon: Soul

I am in love for the first time. I have finally – at *long* last – found my soulmate. I've read Shakespeare, studied Pre-Raphaelite paintings and watched every single episode of *Blind Date*. I feel as though I've been looking for love for an eternity and kissed all the frogs in the world without any major stirrings in my soul. And finally, it's here. The moment to end all moments. The reason for my being, for all of our being, for humanity itself. Love. I've been waiting *forever* for the universe to send me love, this emotion that reminds me how small I am, so insignificant, yet how endless and miraculous at the same time. The thing that Neruda was getting at. The centre of the painting. The top note of a Beethoven symphony. That place only Cilla Black truly understood. I am, of course, in my very early twenties. I'm living in a house-share in Brockley south-east London, my room is next to my best friend Joy's room. Both of us have boyfriends in our bedrooms. I've lit some candles, tealights from the market, and Marcus and I are kissing in the way that young people do – with our entire bodies as opposed to just our mouths. It is then that I first feel it. At first it's simply a sense of change. Something shifting. Then overwhelming desire, and the sense that *everything* has suddenly changed. The colours are brighter. Technicolour. Everything glows orange liquid. A thousand flashing stars. The back of my head feels as if it is being pulled away from my body, making more room inside my mind for these new and overwhelming and desperate feelings and longing.

I must be in love. I am in love.

The world changes focus. Time pauses. The earth stops spinning and it feels as if I'm flying. The scene becomes dreamlike, and nothing, *nothing*, is more important than this one moment. My heartbeat pulses softly in my throat, butterfly wings, and Marcus kisses it as though he is trying to taste the blood through my skin. Surely, on my death bed, this will be the memory to flash before my eyes. My arms and legs wind around Marcus's until it's impossible to imagine that we might ever disentangle. This is forever. Everything is so warm and bright I think my heart will burst from my mouth. The room glows, I glow, and Marcus's skin flashes silver.

Perhaps all of life is contained in this one moment. This breathtaking, mind-bending, body-on-fire feeling. Real love burns. And there is only now.

And then I notice.

A flash of gold. A rising orange. The smell of real burning. Perhaps it is the chemical smell of plastic that jolts me out of my state into reality. Whatever it is that snaps me back I am in the real world once more. I am no longer nymph-like but awkward, and our limbs are stuck at odd angles, my breathing is crackling, and I cough.

We separate, sit up and jump up and back in a moment. It is not love that made me warm and glow golden and feel burning.

My quilt is on fire.

I scream. Marcus screams. Joy runs in and screams, her boyfriend runs in behind her and screams. The fact that the quilt is polyester makes the scene all the more dramatic; it goes up in a ball of flame. Nobody moves. We watch the burning. Then Joy bolts into action, opens the window as wide as it will go, grabs the one corner of the quilt that has yet to ignite, and chucks the quilt out into the navy blue night. It drops from the third floor of our bedrooms straight to the ground, a burning comet, whooshing and further igniting with the oxygen. We run to watch it as it lands, a giant orange fireball, sizzling on the ground. My landlord, who lives in the same house, is drinking a cup of tea in the living room on the ground floor, when the burning material falls past the window. He shouts, his voice carrying through the house to reach us at the top. *What the fuck.* And then, *Christie!* The front door opens, and slams, and we see him, tea still in hand, standing in the garden in front of the quilt, a mini bonfire. He looks up, and we jump away from sight.

Then, a few seconds of silence.

'I thought I was in love,' I say. 'Everything was warm and glowed orange. I felt so hot. Hotter than ever before. I honestly thought it was love.'

The room still feels hot, as if holding a memory of fire – or love. I don't know whether to cry, or to laugh. The men do not laugh. But Joy turns and stares at me for the longest time, before laughing so hard she has to hold her belly. Her body convulses and she leans on the window frame to stay upright. Tears run down her cheeks. I begin to laugh too. We giggle and splutter and burst out cry-laughing. We neither of us pay any attention to our boyfriends gathering their clothes and slinking off. Marcus turns before leaving the room. 'You're mad,' he says. And that makes us laugh even more.

'Quilt on fire,' says Joy. 'I love you, Christie Watson.'

Love has always fascinated me, this thing that exists which you can't see, or touch, or hear, or taste, yet still understand as our single reason for being. Yet it's confusing too. Romantic love is, in my case, a tricky, elusive idea. But I've always been searching for something. During my teens I am searching for acceptance. I spend teenage summers with my paternal grandmother in Mablethorpe, a place the poet, Alfred, Lord Tennyson, also spent childhood summers: *Gray sand banks and pale sunsets – dreary wind; Dim shores, dense rains, and heavy-clouded sea*. My grandmother is a tiny, bird-like woman, who is kind, and collects cacti. She is a spiritualist, 'one foot in this world, and one foot in the next', and is prone to describing the spirits she can see around me, that are wafting around my body, telling me I have 'the gift'. I do not really want the gift. I want to sneak out with my cousins and head to the funfair and flirt with boys – the lads who have dirty hands and look at my cousins and me with direct, unblinking gazes, and give us free rides on the waltzers in exchange for smoky kisses. My grandmother pops up one day, as we sit on the waltzers, messing around with the workers, her head framed with white hair suddenly leaning over the side of our car. She glances at my own recently dyed blue hair and cheap choker necklace covered in skulls, my cousin's boob tube and short shorts, and her eyes are unable to land. There is too much teenage to focus on one bit. 'I'll pray for you,' she says, and then she is gone.

I'm not sure why she is praying for us, or what exactly we have done wrong, and I'm too busy being fourteen to care that much. But I do think a lot at this age about prayer, and Gods and Heaven and Hell and The Universe and Blue Hair Dye. I describe myself as agnostic, the word – I recite – 'derived from the ancient Greek for *without knowledge*, first used in 1869 by Thomas Henry Huxley in a speech at a meeting of the Metaphysical Society – an exclusive (and exclusively male) debating club – to describe his philosophy, which rejects all claims of spiritual or mystical knowledge'. I complain about the outrageous unfairness of patriarchal structures allowing such a club to exist only for men, as though women don't have interesting thoughts. I tell everyone about my agnostic nature too. But, of course, I believe in everything.

In the centre of the graveyard next to my school is an old yew tree, beautiful and creepy, and full of legends. It is *fact* that if you run around that yew tree backwards thirteen times you will invoke evil spirits. We long for these supernatural certainties, a validation of our bizarre ideas. One night three friends and I sleep in my bedroom, sardined into sleeping bags pulled all the way up so my mum can't tell we are fully clothed when she says goodnight. The thrill of doing something exciting and forbidden moves around my body with my blood, filling me up until my skin is clammy. At 3 a.m. the alarm shakes us awake and we creep out into the moonlight. Full moon, naturally. Passing grey-blue clouds. We walk to the church. I have no idea, looking back, what possessed us to want to invoke evil spirits and hang around a graveyard; it felt like something close to a dare, but perhaps it was deeper than that, some kind of proof of our selves. A mysterious external place, mirroring our mysterious internal worlds. We four often talk each other into seeing and believing things until we do, wishing it so hard until it simply is. There is a portal between two worlds, this one and the evil one, which can be accessed by running around a tree; of that we are now completely convinced. We have all seen and heard ghosts from that world, sometimes at the same time. Shared psychotic disorder or induced delusional disorder remains to this day omitted from the DSM manual for psychiatric disorders, but it's well documented. Folie à deux, or folie à quatre in our case, is described as symptoms of shared delusional belief, and sometimes hallucinations, which are transmitted from one individual to another. We are at the age where we share: lipgloss, Slush Puppies, cigarettes – which we spray with perfume, for added chemicals – clothes, eyeliner, Hooch, secrets and irrationality.

We begin to run. I can see us now. Gangly, skinny teen girls, our knees the widest part of our legs, trying awkwardly to run backwards, laughing so hard at the same time. I miss that laughter that spurts out of teen mouths when they are risk-taking with friends. The hysteria of the teen-age. But I do wonder now what would have happened had anyone been in the churchyard that night. My adult brain sees all sorts of danger. But the only danger we see then is danger from the other side of our world. The one we can't always see but exists alongside us. The one Megan's cat sees clearly, when we watch her freeze and back out of a room, looking at something above our heads. A spirit for sure.

We laugh and run, laugh and run. Running backwards is not easy but we make it to ten, eleven, twelve times. A large cloud passes over the moon. And just as we are about to start another circuit, the laughter stops and our hearts race with the enormity of what we are doing. You can feel the change in the air, a heaviness, a sudden humidity loaded with threat. The whites of our eyes flash at each other. We are doing it. Really doing it. Four girls from Stevenage are making witchcraft history and will prove the existence of the afterlife, and create a terrible, violent portal for spirits to enter and liven up our endlessly boring town. And then, at the final hurdle, Megan falls, tripping over a tree root, screaming out in pain. She lies on the ground, clutching her ankle, and we crowd around her, watching her face change shape into agony. But instead of comforting Megan, we all look at each other as the clouds pass by and the moon lights up the graveyard, now covered in low lying fog, and eerier than ever before. 'The twelfth time,' said Amanda. 'The twelfth time around.' The enormity of the timing *just before the thirteenth time* hit our receptive brains and we know. We absolutely know. That someone out there, *up there*, is protecting us from ourselves.

After that we throw ourselves into the spiritual world with gusto. We practise tarot, wrapping our cards in silk for protection. I wear a small necklace of the evil eye and I line my window with dreamcatchers. We read each others' thoughts, and try and levitate one another off the ground. We collect crystals and we burn cedar, filling the room with smoke. My teenage bedroom stinks. Sage, incense, anointing oil, Body Shop Vanilla Musk. We hold séances, never quite working out who is moving the dial to spell the word MURDERED and never quite questioning why all spirits we contact are serial killers and dangerous psychopaths, instead of grandfatherly types who smoke pipes and have sheds and slippers and allotments.

Alongside trying to invoke evil spirits, and my interest in superstition and paganism and mysticism and telepathy and crystal balls and healing hands, I become a bit obsessed with organised religions too. I wear a St Christopher necklace and, at around the age of fourteen, the peak of my awfulness, begin to pray. But instead of praying for thanks – or indeed forgiveness – I rant about the ozone layer, and the life expectancy being so low in some countries, basically telling God off for global failures. I read the Bible, not to absorb wisdom, but to edit, imagining the words better placed, the imagery more vivid. I quickly bore of Christianity. Catholics seem more certain of everything and I like the rules and the rosary beads, but a girl in my music school is Catholic and has terrible acne, despite all the Hail Marys. Maybe Sikhism is for me? I like the red bracelet. But then, I like the Ganesh statues of Hinduism. Buddhism? I like the idea of Sting and tantric sex. I try on religions like new clothes, every week claiming I am something else. I search the Quran and Torah and Bhagavad Gita and then read *The Celestine Prophecy* by James Redfield so many times I can recite passages. *The First Insight is an awareness of the mysterious occurrences that change one's life, the feeling that some other process is operating.*

My eyes are permanently half-closed, scanning the world for coincidences. I think of my nan and the phone rings. It's my nan! I dream of a rail accident, then there is one on the news! I listen to Gospel music and visit temples. I study astrology and the Chinese zodiac and often excuse bad behaviour by simply shouting to my mum: Virgo! Year of the Dragon! I do a paper round on which I find myself a Jehovah's Witness boyfriend who I am desperate to talk to about spirituality, but who just wants to dry hump me, once, leaving a patch of jizz on my jeans.

I cared for a woman during my early nursing years who was totally convinced that an alien had abducted her, hollowed out her insides, including her organs, lasered her back together and left her here on earth, with nothing at all in her centre. I remember how we focused on her delusions, her psychosis, on convincing her that she was safe, with organs where they should be. I told her that UFOs do not exist, and reiterated that she is very unwell, but will get better. I can't remember us spending too much time on the word she kept repeating: hollow. On what that might signify. Symptoms – in her case severe psychosis – are not necessarily cause, they are sometimes treatment for cause. Her intellectualisation that her feeling of emptiness had an explanation – irrational or not – gave her some comfort. She could visualise why she felt so bare and desolate. 'Be careful telling her that UFOs don't exist,' the psychiatrist told me. Insight, in her case, I was told, might be a dangerous thing. 'Symptoms might not be a sign of illness at all, but a sign of wellness trying to treat the illness.'

Now I am the one who feels hollow. Emptied out. My insides missing. At forty-two, seemingly perimenopausal, I find myself searching again, and with something like urgency, for answers. I feel as if I have never known less about everything. I listen to the astronaut Scott Kelly talking about looking at the earth from space. He describes increasingly noticing things that he didn't see before. The earth has a layer, like a contact lens over an eyeball, upon which we completely depend, the atmosphere, while the earth also has patches of brown, giant patches of pollution, that are new. I am increasingly noticing things I didn't see before: my fragility, vulnerability, the patches of brown. I'm now at a vantage point, almost midlife, where I should surely and clearly be able to see the before and after with clarity and understanding, but I can't make sense of it all.

Instead of finding meaning, I'm crying in a church. All my emotions feel too big to contain; my sobs escape and echo around the building. I don't know what has prompted this, or even my slipping into the empty church on the way home, but I am overwhelmed, seeking sanctuary. At the front of the church are dozens of candles, which people have lit to remember loved ones. I light four and watch the tiny flames. I sit on the pew at the front and try to focus on the stained glass. The smell of the benches reminds me of the smell of my dad's jumper: woodsmoke and oranges and polish. Everything feels cold and draughty, but my body and my head are burning. A woman is cleaning, and half-watching me, a look of pity moves across her face then is gone. She's seen too many people crying, perhaps. 'You OK?' she walks over and hovers, polish in one hand and cloth in the other. She is older than me, maybe in her sixties, and has short grey hair that looks as if it has been cut using a bowl, the haircut of early childhood.

'Not really,' I say.

She nods, knowingly. Then smiles. Something about her smile makes me stop crying at once. 'None of us are, not really. But at least we are in it together. Would you like to pray, maybe?'

I notice then that she is wearing a clerical collar, and maybe has all the answers that I don't. But I'm too embarrassed to tell her that I'm not sure I've ever believed in prayer, and I'm unsure God exists. I fiercely hold on to the idea of empirical reality, but have nothing to believe in, not least myself. As a teenager who believed in everything, I now find myself increasingly cynical, rolling my eyes at the notion of angels, or chakras, or depictions of heaven and hell.

Nonetheless, the words spill out of me. 'I keep remembering all the people I've seen take a final breath. And they're accumulating, these memories. I think all the time about my dad taking his final breath. I'm stuck in that single memory of him, as though the screen has frozen.'

The woman sits down, next to me but not too close, and we watch the miniature candles burn for a while. It's pin-drop-quiet and still. 'I thought by my age I'd have some answers,' I tell her. 'But life makes no sense at all. I just thought everything would be different by now. I feel like I know even less every day. I mean, I thought I'd have it together by now. I don't understand why we're here. What life means. What love means. I thought I'd have it all sorted out. Other people seem to. Other women. I'm seeing a therapist, who thinks it could all be down to hormones. But that doesn't feel right, you know?'

She smiles and then says, 'The profound mysteries of life. We don't find any answers as we get older. Only more questions.'

I look to her for answers, but she has none, though she appears happy with that state. Despite my increasing doubts, I've always admired people of faith. I wonder if our relationship with faith, as well as love, changes shape as we age. My dad was an out-and-out atheist. But when he was dying he was won over by a local vicar who used to visit and drink whisky with him, laughing in the living room until the late hours.

When he announced he was planning his funeral in a church, my mum, brother and I were more than a little shocked. And although he claimed it was more for Mum than for him, I did wonder if Dad was losing his scepticism, or if he was afraid, or even hopeful. As a parent of a child who I looked after once told me: *faith is not knowing, it's hoping.*

Maybe love too is not knowing, it's hoping.

'Before my dad died he wrote this beautiful piece that I read at his funeral. Love each other, he wrote. It's the only thing that matters, in the end. Love.'

She nods. 'I agree.'

I nod too. But never once did I imagine at the age that I am, almost at the midpoint, that I would still be confused and baffled by love. And faith. And life, and humanity. 'I have no idea what anything means,' I say. 'I'm not making sense. I have no idea why I'm here crying in church. Why I'm crying all the time. My emotions are all over the place.'

She pauses a while. Then, 'I found it a time of reflection,' she says. 'My forties. Maybe the most important time to re-evaluate what we think and who we are. And just to let you know, nobody has it together. None of us.' She smiles again. 'Sounds like your therapist is giving you good advice.'

Luisa is cross-legged on a wing-backed chair opposite me. She has her hands folded gently on her lap, in an open posture. I wonder if psychotherapists learn how to sit, because surely their body language must be part of the process. One of the most excruciating aspects of therapy, for me, is the silence, and how much learning to sit in the silence feels like work. I hate sitting in silence. I've tried meditating over the years, and only ever managed to produce more thoughts, filling my head instead of emptying it. I want to fill the space, make it feel less empty, break up awkwardness with conversation. Every time I try to meditate, I sit cross-legged and close my eyes, but instead of a peaceful revelation dawning, thoughts explode: *Did I answer that urgent email? Is it someone's birthday? Do knees sag?*

The inside of my mouth feels crunchy, full of grit. Of course, the feelings I have about hating the silence in these sessions are telling me something important. Being uncomfortable is hard for me. I resort to humour. I am like a small child, hiding from something I don't understand. Here in this therapy room there is only my story, and nowhere to hide. I realise that I'm vulnerable, exposed, and I hate that. But although she doesn't reach out her arms, I feel as though Luisa is holding me, and I am fluid and she is steady and solid. She is a bucket and I am water. It feels like I'm dancing around and skittish, although my body is perfectly still. The choreography between us is complex: Luisa sits in silence until I break, often I repeat something I've already said. I apologise a lot. I ramble. I glance at the wave picture. Make another joke. Try and fix my eyes on hers until they sting, both of us knowing I'm desperate to look away. My body comes to the rescue. My stomach gurgles loud enough that she jumps and we both smile. 'You're processing things,' she says. 'Did you see the GP yet?'

I shake my head. 'I have an appointment next week. But I'm really not convinced this is simply hormones...'

She frowns a fraction. 'Nothing is simply one thing or another. But it feels like a positive step to get checked.'

There is quiet for a while, and I stare at the picture. My eye twitches.

'Does it make you feel anything, that painting?'

I shrug. I don't know how to tell her I feel like I'm drowning all the time. Or perhaps that I want to drown. My stomach rumbles again.

'Our bodies process things before our minds,' she says. Sometimes she'll say things like this that sound so 'woowoo' I find it hard to listen, now that, seemingly, I believe in nothing unprovable. Joy is into crystals and Reiki and believes in all things mystical. When I phone her in crisis, she sends me miniature Guatemalan worry dolls to put underneath my pillow. I thank her, but smirk a bit, and stash them in my bedside cabinet. I like hard facts, science, medicine and intellectualisation. But the more I sit with Luisa, the more I do listen to my body. It is speaking. 'What drew you to nursing?'

The question surprises me. What has that got to do with

feeling so desperate? I give her my stock answer, the career ideas I went through, my flighty nature, how it balanced out my chaos, and suited my love of the idea of structure, of cleanliness, order.

'And why children's intensive care? It seems like a place of great suffering.' I think a while. A good part of my life has been working in children's intensive care, where impossibly small, broken bodies reminded me daily that tragedy is everywhere. But it's also a place where, despite tragedy, there is always hope. We talk a while about the work, the nature of it. I remember the children I cared for over the years who stood out the most. What I remember about them is not their physicality or their bodies, but their spirits, characters, personalities. Their sheer will and determination. The falling apart of my own body feels ridiculous and superficial. I am not ill. Perimenopause is not a disease. In *Illness as Metaphor*, Susan Sontag describes illness as 'the night side of life, a more onerous citizenship. Everyone who is born holds dual citizenship, in the kingdom of the well and in the kingdom of the sick. Although we all prefer to use the good passport, sooner or later each of us is obliged, at least for a spell, to identify ourselves as citizens of that other place.' I am enormously lucky to have spent most of my life, thus far, in the Kingdom of the Well. The absurdity and vanity of my worries against the real and present pain of genuine illness is a place of uncomfortable privilege. An itchy, ill-fitting coat. 'I am ashamed of how I'm feeling,' I say. 'There really is nothing wrong with me so it almost feels as if I'm finding things or focusing on minutiae. I mean, woe is me, I am single at midlife and have grey pubic hair... But other women in the world appear to be doing love and life better and with more dignity: there seems to be an army of middle-aged polished women, smiling and embracing wellness and chamomile tea, sailing through their forties and fifties with soy beans and stable, happy relationships. And I find myself in the giant fish finger freezer in the supermarket.'

She almost smiles, but catches it just in time. 'And who even rambles on like this in a therapy session?' I close my mouth before any other words spill out.

But she doesn't ask about any of what I've just voiced. 'It feels like an interesting choice you made, to go and work in a place of extreme suffering.' She pauses, waits while I think.

'You're right. I wonder what draws people to do such extreme jobs.'

'Perhaps,' she says, 'when we help others who suffer, we can forget about our own pain, for a while.'

Silence. Maybe in some cases. I think of some of my colleagues. How they like hard facts too. The language of medicine is protective of the clinician, a division of sorts, a separation of us and them. Us and us might be a truism, but is maybe too terrifying a prospect when work is with tragedy. Clinicians hide behind Latin, or in acronyms, or long technical sentences that are hard to unpick, and too often hide death in euphemisms: *passed away, gone, passed on,* perhaps lest we confront the prospect of our own mortality. That we will all die is never more explicit than in an intensive care unit. It is the hum in the background.

Luisa is still the bucket and I am the water in this room. But perhaps it is more than that. The room is the sea and Luisa and I are both in it, holding our breath and diving for clues.

We sit in the silence, in the water, a while.

I'm not exactly suffering. I had a happy childhood, up until my teen years. I had loving parents, was safe, had a home and food, and now, as a white, able-bodied woman, with a job and a home, and living in the UK, I'm coated with privilege. An extra thick skin of luck and circumstance.

'Comparative suffering is not helpful. We can't measure our suffering against someone else's,' she says.

We can, I think. Nurses do it all the time. There is always somebody worse off than me; nursing has taught me that. But I do agree that people approach life, and change, in wildly different ways.

'I don't think my choice to become a nurse in children's intensive care was about suffering,' I say, 'it was the people around me. My brilliant colleagues. I so enjoyed learning from older and wiser women.' I stop on that a while. 'One of the things I've always loved,' I say, 'is being around much older and much wiser women.'

She nods. 'And now you are becoming one.'

I don't feel very wise. But I'm definitely searching for wisdom about love, life and the universe. I look for verity in books, both non-fiction and fiction. Non-fiction, it seems to me, contains fact, and yet fiction is truth. I want to interrogate this notion, my distorted state of reality pushing me to question what is real or not real, to understand in any case what is contained in the Book of Wisdom: the circuits of years, the position of stars. I look to other women for answers. I have no interest in the wellness brigade. I read an article in which Gwyneth Paltrow explains her response to perimenopause: recalibrating her fitness regimen, a clean-eating diet comprised of whole foods, such as leafy greens and lean, ethically sourced protein. 'I do a panel every six months now to ensure that everything is aligned.' I have no idea what this panel is that she's doing, and I have just eaten an entire pack of chocolate Hobnobs. I try and absorb wisdom from writers I admire. Julia Samuel, a psychotherapist, writes in *This Too Shall Pass*: 'The menopause represents a step into another phase of life. It is the physical embodiment of no longer being fertile. Sexuality, fertility and motherhood are a key part of a woman's identity and perceived societal purpose. Therefore, finding a way to carve a new identity and purpose can give renewed meaning to her life.' I spend hours in bookshops and libraries, always my sanctuary, and find books that speak to my situation indirectly, but directly too. In the poetic and illuminating meditation on menopause, *Flash Count Diary*, American writer Darcey Steinke searches too for meaning: 'Freedom is on the horizon – freedom from child care and domestic duties, from trying to be beautiful, and the leering male gaze, from derailing sexual desires.' I don't feel free. More caged in, closed, locked away. I find many books in the library. But my concentration is poor and my brain fog heavy and so, after a few minutes of reading, I wander around pulling old books off the shelves, the dustier the better, and smell them. A librarian watches me. 'Is there anything in the world that smells better than old books?' I say, and she raises her eyebrows. She's around a decade or so younger than me, and I feel like warning her that she too might be walking around soon enough, as eccentric as I am, unable to read books so smelling them instead. 'It's a comfort surrounding myself with books by women who are making sense of things.' She frowns, and nods at this, as though she finally understands me.

My search for wisdom takes me to unexpected places. When I am asked to break a window at Harvey Nichols to commemorate a hundred years since the suffrage won the vote for most women, I feel like I've arrived. *This* is how I imagined my forties. Not standing in a fish finger freezer. Powerful, feminist, world-changing. I am standing next to Helen Pankhurst, the great granddaughter of Emeline Pankhurst, carrying a crowbar, ready to smash up the patriarchy. I can feel the sagacity floating off her skin, and landing on mine. Simply standing near her surely makes me a better person. There are dozens of photographers, and twelve women from many sectors all stand waiting to walk past them and break the glass. We have forfeited the protective eyewear. We are dangerous, confident women. I am so desperately trying to make best friends with Helen Pankhurst that she stands back a little, and frowns. 'Are you OK?' she asks.

And I realise I've been smiling, sycophantic. I lower my smile. Shrug as if it's every day I get to stand next to the descendant of one of the heroes of feminism. A woman who must be so full of wisdom you can probably smell it in the air around her. I am regretting spraying all the perfume testers in Harvey Nichols, after getting here early. She coughs. I do not smell wise. I lift my head and raise the crowbar, nod at the photographers in front of the window we are about to shatter. 'Let's get ready to strut,' I say.

And Helen looks at me, with something like pity. 'March. We don't strut. We women march.'

*

While I am crying in a church looking for spiritual answers to the location and nature of my soul, to the meaning of love, and ageing and wisdom, my friend Orla is formulating what she calls a Fuck It Bucket List – her very own brand of HRT: *It is not in medication that I'll be looking for lost joy*. Her husband left her three years ago for a model who is twenty-five years his junior and Orla recently heard that he has had a pole fitted in the living room of his purpose-built flat, so that his girlfriend can practise her pole dancing at home. 'This is the man who used to sit at Heathrow airport for days on end watching planes and recording on a spreadsheet the exact times they took off and landed.' She laughs but there is a sadness that surrounds her. Her husband had never wanted children, and she had grudgingly accepted that. And now his pole-dancing model girlfriend is pregnant and he is apparently delighted. This is a sad story and, even sadder, it's one that I've heard numerous times. Orla is fighting the melancholy with practical responses. Her bucket list is ever growing. She adds to it almost daily: aerial trapeze, Torture Gardens, hiking in the fjords of Norway, tattoos, hot yoga, whisky tour of Scotland, an ayahuasca retreat. 'What else?' she asks. 'What can I add?' But I have nothing: I admire her chutzpah but have no inclination of my own to jump out of a plane, cycle from John O'Groats to Land's End or run an ultramarathon. These days, even popping to the shop to buy milk feels momentous.

'There is a sense that death is closing in,' Orla says. 'We're at an age where it's ever present. We can't just sit around waiting. Now is the time.'

She's right, of course. As a teenager, I couldn't imagine being mortal, but now I hear stories all the time of dying friends. People I love are falling away. They come in a hurry, these tragedies. I lose a friend in an air crash, another to a stroke, another to cancer. A friend dies by suicide, and a young relative from a heart attack. Life is too short. It's a truth that is both scary and liberating. Every single day matters, and the monotony of life seems bizarre, even ludicrous. Worrying seems frivolous. 'Too many lives are surely a waste,' Orla continues. 'Sleepwalking towards death.' But then she looks sad again. 'I can't believe she's pregnant.' Her eyes are hard and angry and there's a frown cutting between them. 'My periods have stopped completely. I wonder why it is, that our periods stop?'

I think a lot about that, the meaning of infertility. What is it for? What does it mean, this transformation, this profound change? This 'change of life' is deeper than physical, more than a lack of stable hormones. Hormone replacement therapy is a good answer for many women, and it's something I plan to ask my GP about, but I wonder if it's the answer to a superficial question. There's something about women at midlife when they become aware of something within themselves that is ocean deep and near impossible to reach. It becomes a time of almost forced soul-searching. In her aptly titled essay, 'Philosophical Plumbing', Mary Midgley argued that philosophy is like plumbing – nobody notices it until it goes wrong. 'Then suddenly we become aware of some bad smells, and we have to take up the floorboards and look at the concepts of even the most ordinary piece of thinking.'

It is time to take up the floorboards.

The universe is surely questioning midlife women, whispering something important about humanity, what it means to be human. Humans are one of only five creatures who go through and live beyond the menopause. The others are all whales: orcas, short-finned pilot whales, belugas, narwhals. Women and whales. Mystical, magical creatures, full of the secrets written in stars. Whales, too, have the ability to experience deep-rooted emotional suffering. They also have the capacity to feel love. Patrick Hof and Estel Van Der Gucht of the New York Consortium in Evolutionary Primatology spent fifteen years studying the brains of orcas and other large whales, and found spindle cells. These spindle cells were found in the area of the brain that regulates emotional functions such as social organisation, empathy, speech, intuition and rapid gut reactions in humans. These are the cells that allow humans to feel love. And *rapid gut reactions*. My spindle cells must have been out of control or off or misunderstood or misfiring ever since I set my duvet alight. Maybe now, finally, is the time to regulate them? Maybe the run up to menopause *is* a time for reflection about all things, and about rebalancing priorities. Maybe this is a time to reset and work out what I want from life? Or at least, need.

And I hear my dad's words on repeat: *Love each other. Love is the only thing that matters, in the end.*

I hear Luisa's words too. *You are becoming a wiser, older woman too.*

I don't feel wise at all. But I want to find meaning, now more than ever. I have no answers at all. I don't understand life. I don't understand love. I have no idea what it means to be human. Or even who I am. But the perimenopause, the rocky road to the middle, the centre point, is surely the time to examine what it's all for. Despite lack of real illness, I'm identifying as a citizen of another place, and it's not a gradual easing, from the Kingdom of the Young, to the Kingdom of the Old. Who I have been, and who I am becoming, consumes me. My identity becomes less clear every day. But there's one thing I'm certain of:

I want my quilt on fire.

3

Je T'aime: Body

The GP is a young woman with a bright smile. She is wearing Louboutins, I notice, which seems an odd choice for work attire in a primary care practice in a dirty south London street, the waiting room of which is stuffed full of the great unwashed. The room is standard NHS GP: a plastic chair (wipeable) facing out next to a desk so you can't see your own information on the computer screen unless the GP turns the screen. A strange power imbalance. A blood pressure machine, next to a phone. On the opposite wall a thin bed (also wipeable) and a crappy thin curtain that never properly closes. Next to that, a trolley, of sorts, containing gloves, glucose testing strips, speculums and swabs. A sink at the end has a rolled-up supply of plastic aprons above it, and wall-mounted boxes of more gloves in different sizes and colours.

'How can I help?' She doesn't look up from the computer. My GP friend tells me they are more like Citizens Advice Bureaux than clinicians these days. 'I spend a lot of my day talking about housing, writing sick notes or discussing debt in relation to depression. Social illness is a huge part of what we deal with now. Suffering medical symptoms of emotional and societal disease.' He has moved to another town as his patients kept accosting him in the street, asking for money, or advice or food or, on one occasion, if he wanted to buy a kidney. Another GP colleague tells me she writes notes on prescriptions, as well as, or sometimes instead of the actual prescription: *I see you. I am sorry you are going through this. It will get better. It is not your fault.* She says her patients keep the prescriptions, one on his fridge, another underneath her pillow. 'I feel as if we're living in a time when these words and this communication and compassion sometimes have as much effect as the medicine. Our medicine no longer fits our diseases. People are suffering existentially.'

I'm suffering existentially, and as if I'm wasting my GP's time. And it's hard to get into words what is happening. Is there a language for this? 'I'm feeling very low. Anxious. Not sleeping. I saw a therapist and she suggested I get my hormones checked as it might be perimenopause. I'm only forty-two.'

She flashes me a look. Another smile. Pity. I remember being a teen and my parents throwing a party for a neighbour turning forty. I can distinctly remember being totally dumbstruck as to why you'd want to celebrate that. How old forty is. How close to death. I couldn't imagine ever becoming a woman in my forties. The thought of it made my stomach turn, as though the idea of middle age was curdled milk. The GP smiles again and flicks her hair. She can't imagine growing towards middle age either, I suspect, despite her job. I wonder how many people have sat on this plastic seat and tried to explain their suffering. Hospital doctors get all the acclaim yet it is here in the shabby, rundown GP clinics where the most lives are saved. It's just not very glamorous. Maybe that's why the Louboutins.

She tells me the facts. The highest suicide rate in the UK among women is currently forty-five to forty-nine. Peak sadness hits us at forty-seven years. 'Menopause has been known to exacerbate bipolar disorder, and perimenopause may increase the risk of first presentation psychosis: schizophrenia, for example, typically has its onset in young adulthood, but there is a second peak in women around menopause.'

'I am five years away from peak sadness?' I ask. I can't feel any sadder. 'I've peaked already.' I also have brain fog, insomnia, anxiety, depression, mood swings, fatigue, memory loss, dissociation, migraines, emotions, mood, memory, rage, lack of motivation, as well as the sadness, or emptiness, all of which, I discover, are symptoms of perimenopause. I also have many of the physical symptoms she then lists: hot flushes; night sweats; vaginal dryness; headaches; palpitations; discomfort during sex; vaginal atrophy; dizziness; recurrent urinary tract infections; incontinence; irregular periods; bladder problems;

osteoporosis; increased cholesterol; decreased libido; bleeding gums; hair loss; dry skin, hair, nails, vagina, eyes, mouth; joint pain; decreased vision; fatigue; muscle pain; breast tenderness; numb hands and feet.

'People focus on the well-known physical symptoms of perimenopause, the hot flushes, for example, but the symptoms are largely neurological, and can lead to neurological decline, degenerative disease even. Oestrogen is a master regulator...'

Neurological decline? Neurodegenerative disease? Peak sadness? And are the physical symptoms well known? My GP – unlike, I will discover later, too many GPs – is well informed about perimenopause. But in many cases, in my case, even as a healthcare professional I had no idea about these symptoms. No clue.

I once read a quote, I believe from Khalil Gibran: *he who tries to separate the body from the mind or the mind from the body distances his heart from the truth.* I am far from the truth. But I try to describe what I'm experiencing to the GP anyway. 'Suddenly my mind and body feel completely separate, working independently, falling apart in different ways.'

She nods, knowingly. 'Then there are the social factors,' she says. 'Because clearly that list is not long enough for women.' She laughs, and flicks her hair again.

My hair is falling out.

I think about when it first happened, and the handful of

loosening hair whenever I wash it. My scalp becoming visible. My friends say they cannot notice, but I suspect they are being kind. I'm now unable to brush my hair, as even something like gentle brushing causes small clumps to fall away. I no longer wear black, to avoid seeing so clearly the wispy strands of hair constantly falling out onto my shoulders. I have started looking at other women's hair with great envy. At younger photos of myself with better hair. Of course, in the grand scheme of life, hair loss should be trivial. But it doesn't feel trivial. The word trivial means very common and therefore inconsequential, but it originates from the word 'crossroads'.

'Ageing parents,' she says, 'teen children, financial stress.' She smiles at me, looks up from the screen. 'Think of it less as losing youth,' she says, 'but gaining wisdom.'

I look at her without blinking.

'What are my options?' I ask her. I have no idea if she can help me, and how, or even if medication is the way forward, but there's one thing I understand for sure: I clearly need regulating.

And she looks suddenly older than her years, and wiser. 'HRT,' she says.

In 1865 Francis Skae, an assistant medical officer of the Borough Asylum in Birmingham wrote about 'climacteric insanity in women'. Skae describes the women suffering depression of spirits, sleeplessness, restlessness, fear of undefined evil and inattention to ordinary domestic affairs, all of which can lead to melancholia.

I recognise all of these symptoms. I have no energy for anything, least of all 'domestic affairs'. How many women were burned as witches? Or locked up in lunatic asylums? Women were locked away, or given treatments ranging from opium to marijuana, to herbal remedies. The suggested treatments for women at midlife varied wildly around the world. In some cultures, nature was turned to as a solution to a natural process. Chinese herbal medicine has been used for centuries to help relieve the symptoms of menopause – and continues to be used, in Chinese public hospitals, for example. Native American herbal treatments included alfalfa, chasteberry, dong quia, maca, oak, sage, red clover, star anise and sweetgrass. Meanwhile, in England women were 'treated' with vaginal injections and testicular juice, bloodletting and a concoction of lead, morphine and chloroform. Surgery, including ovariotomies and cliterodectomies, became increasingly common in America. When I compare my situation to women throughout history, I should feel lucky. I hear whispers of my ancestors, chastising me: *look what we went through. Look how far women have come.* But of course, the circumstances of women have not come far enough, and it has not been fast enough.

Women continue to have conversations that start, 'Can you believe we are still having this conversation?'

Medical interest in the menopause increased considerably in the mid-nineteenth century, and in the 1930s people starting describing it as a deficiency disease. The fight about HRT goes on. 'All post-menopausal women are castrates,' Robert A. Wilson wrote in 1968, in his bestselling book *Feminine Forever*. 'But, with HRT, a woman's breasts and genital organs will not shrivel. She will be much more pleasant to live with and will not become dull and unattractive'. Wilson, a British-born gynaecologist, subsequently found to be sponsored by an HRT drug company, was described as the 'Hugh Hefner of the menopause' by Sandra Coney. In her book, *The Menopause Industry*, she says: 'menopause is a natural part of life, not an illness, and it doesn't necessarily require medical intervention.' This was not a new idea, even if a quiet one. In 1936 Marie Stopes argued that the crises of a woman's life have been much descanted upon by male medical writers – and perhaps the most artificially created has been her 'change'.

I am changing. And it doesn't feel at all natural or evolutionary. I think of my peers, my friends of the same age also suffering. We are a club, I realise. And so many of us have less confidence than before: perhaps unresolved trauma resurfaces and refuses to be ignored around the time of menopause. Many of my friends, too, are fighting an unknown enemy, thrashing around in their own psyches. Emma is the woman who would clamber up onto stages at gigs and high-five the band. Now, however, she speaks quietly, in a shaky voice, and has found she can't stop crying either. Others are experiencing physical manifestations of emotional pain and health anxiety, others are self-sabotaging with harmful behaviours and addictions: alcohol; drugs; cigarettes; difficult relationships with food; one, a sex addiction. Even those who are not suffering in such extreme ways are different. A bit broken.

Joy is famously dramatic and exuberant, the life and soul of a party, always full of joie de vivre, lively, engaged and interested. She has seemingly endless energy, and makes the most of every day, with elaborate plans to buy a piece of woodland and turn it into a 'personal utopia, with a pond for swimming in', or a camper van to explore the wildest parts of the country. She's always busy, with a houseful of laughing children. Giant pots of food bubbling away, hers is the only home I've ever been to where I start salivating on the doorstep, her front garden full of brightly coloured flowers and the smell of brown stew chicken. And despite being the most hardworking woman I know, she is the friend who never forgets a birthday, or to send a thank-you note. She's the type of person to make you feel important, even when she's busy. Joy is beautiful inside and out, and her cup is always half-full, her enthusiasm for life and love and family and friends is infectious. She loves parties and dancing all night and has a wicked sense of humour. She holds court, relaying funny stories until my friends and I are cry-laughing. She loves the limelight and has long been the extrovert of extroverts, and yet recently I've noticed her energy levels changing. She's not at all her usual Miss Giddy Knickers, as we affectionately call her, but is instead more subdued now, somehow quieter, smaller.

'I feel as if I'm wading through sand,' she tells me. 'Every day. My skin is dull. I've lost my shine. I feel so hopeless, and I don't know why.'

Like Emma and Joy I feel I have lost something indefinable. Something is missing. I want my shine back. I want to know the part of myself I have lost, and how I can get it back. I want to gain, not lose. I need the drugs. But still, as my friends tell me, 'it's probably easier to get hold of laudanum, or crack cocaine, than it is to get hold of HRT'.

Luckily my GP ends up being brilliant. 'You'll likely take two or three weeks to feel any effect,' she tells me, tapping her heels on the floor. 'Just change the patch twice a week and let me know if you have any issues.'

'That's it? You don't need to take any more bloods or anything?'

'I'll do routine bloods, as you're younger than forty-five, but essentially that's it,' she says. It's as if she has a secret I don't know about yet.

She tells me that the small transparent patches stick onto

my skin, but if I don't get on with them I can use gel instead. We discuss that HRT is not for everyone but it's suitable for most people. She tells me that there is little to no change in the risk of breast cancer if you take oestrogen-only HRT, and no increased risk of blood clots with the oestrogen-only HRT patches, and as I am planning to have a Mirena coil fitted anyway, this type of HRT is suitable for me. 'But there are many different treatments available to women,' she tells me. 'If HRT is not right, there are non-hormonal medications we could talk about, and other treatments, but most women are able to have HRT, and the benefits outweigh the risks in the vast majority of cases, and actually reduce risks of things like osteoporosis and heart disease. There's no increased risk of breast cancer in women under fifty-one using any type of HRT and it's very low risk for other women.'

Of course – regardless of HRT or alternative treatments, perimenopause is not straightforward or linear. She knows – or suspects – I'll be in to see her repeatedly over the coming years. She understands before I do that I'll be back with a stress fracture, and insomnia and abnormal bleeding, and all the crying and rage. And I'll need to go up and up on my dose. And for me, at least, HRT will provide relief of the physical side of this change. But there is far more than physicality going on here. In any case, she doesn't want to scare me, I suppose. She doesn't mention a shrinking vagina. Maybe menopause is a bit like childbirth. If it were revealed how bad it is, younger women would live in fear. Men would, too.

I'm afraid now. I can't go around this fire, I am walking into it. I feel like my body is failing me but that is, of course, a gross exaggeration. What right do I have to make such a big deal of such insignificant pain? I spent much of my life working as a nurse with people whose bodies had failed them or been damaged in some terrible way. The things I saw as a nurse are hard to describe. We are earthy, us humans, a walking mass of matter that disintegrates. How slowly or quickly depends on how lucky we are, but that disintegration is both universal and inevitable. Having cared for people suffering pain, disease, illness: people with long-term conditions, irrecoverable breathing difficulties; people with damage to internal organs – brains or kidneys or livers; or people with bones that don't work or tumors that do, I have much respect for my own body. Being able to take a walk, breathe deeply, sleep, eat dinner, talk – these are things I'm acutely aware are a privilege that not everybody has. I'd like to say my experiences taught me much about humility. But although I try to be thankful every single day for the way my body works, I feel desperately neurotic: wrong, broken. This is a kind of painful awakening, a reminder of uncertainty, of how little I understand of the universe, and of myself.

The physical symptoms are the most obvious ones, and perhaps the symptoms talked about most openly. I am glad we are speaking about these horrors; it feels almost unbelievable that this process of life that every woman goes though has been, at times, hidden away. But if menopause was about only physical change surely women everywhere would suffer in the same way. Yet physical symptoms and manifestations of the menopause vary around the world. In Japan, it's shoulder pain, while in India, it's poor eyesight; in Costa Rica, women report shortness of breath, while women in UAE report head and neck pain; in China, women have a consistently low chance of experiencing, or perhaps reporting, any symptoms. The mystery of the menopause extends even further than culture, beyond borders. Its origins, and purpose, has some scientists arguing that it is an evolutionary accident, while others claim it is about competition between a mother and her adult daughter, for the most viable offspring, or that 'granny' is now needed to help raise grandchildren. But the granny theory of menopause is discredited by other mammals who do not go through menopause, including elephants, the matriarchs continuing to reproduce, all the while caring for grandchildren too. For every theory, there is a counter-argument. What is it for then, this change?

Judith Gurewich, a publisher and psychoanalyst, writes in a newsletter for Other Press that 'when we lose our mind, our body usually finds it'. I've definitely lost my mind, and my body is fast behind it, my soul and spirit too feel bruised and battered. This is more than biology. 'In examining disease,' Oliver Sacks said in his book *The Man Who Mistook His Wife for a Hat*, 'we gain wisdom about anatomy and physiology and biology. In examining the person with disease we gain wisdom about life.' Of course, perimenopause is not a disease, but a natural process of ageing, though it feels like there is much to examine behind the label. My HRT patch might save me, a bit, yet it resembles a sticking plaster in more than one way. Dressings can sometimes encourage healing. But the wound is usually still there, of course. Underneath. What's inside my skin, I wonder? The factors that influence women's bodies have *always* been more than biology; our physicality is a knotted mass of history, sociology and philosophy and, of course, there is no space more political than a woman's body. Women's bodies everywhere are too often a map of hurt, a landscape of suffering. Perhaps, for some women, for me, perimenopause is an eruption of deep-seated pain. In *The Body Keeps the Score*, Bessel van der Kolk describes how trauma lodges inside us unless resolved. Does perimenopause dislodge it? Is there a possibility that anything buried away demands to be dealt with midlife, if a woman is to live with her whole self? So many friends of my age describe the failings of their bodies but conversely, also the feeling that they no longer care or worry about the things they used to worry about. Maybe we fall apart in order to put ourselves back together in a new way. A surgery of sorts. Traumatic to go through, yet necessary to heal. Whatever the cause of this process, I don't buy that it's simply a period of dwindling oestrogen and progesterone and testosterone, a bouquet of hormone deficiency. Every trauma I've been through in my life seems to be bursting through my blood vessels and bones and settling just below my skin. I can see hurt inside the green-blue veins on my inner forearms. Internal body art.

The word 'oestrogen' is derived from the Greek *oistros* (mad desire) and *gennan* (to produce). As women age, we are more susceptible to cancers that feed off these hormones. Could menopause, then, be about preservation? When we no longer have a need for fertility, are our bodies cleverly removing unnecessary risks? Or are we simply tired of mad desire, finished with it, exhausted by all that it brings? I have no hypothesis. Regardless, I continue to search for meaning in medicine. However, while menopause has long been medicalised in many countries, the medical establishment appears largely unaware of up-to-date scientific research around contemporary treatments. That so many doctors seem so poorly informed about symptoms and diagnosis of perimenopause, and its treatment, including HRT, is shocking.

I search in philosophy. Jungian theory holds that midlife

is key to losing the 'false self' we cling to in youth, towards individuation, a process of self-actualisation; the midlife is an integration of thinking, sensation, feeling and intuition. But if anything, I feel disintegrated. Lacan seems, to me, to speak to midlife more. He argued that what is symbolic is misrecognised as real. For example, unconscious mental conflicts are suffered as bodily afflictions and ailments. Perhaps the perimenopause, a collective turning point, is more abstract than we can imagine or capture in words. Plus, every single woman is different. My mum describes her perimenopause as having been symptomless. I am suspicious of this. But other friends say they have minimal symptoms that are relieved with exercise. My symptoms are extreme and some of them unexplainable. For example, the perimenopause has, weirdly and unexpectedly, resulted in my feet growing a full size bigger. But this is not the first time my feet have grown overnight; nor is it the first time my body has spoken of things my conscious mind has not yet been able to process.

I was one year and five days old when my brother, Tom, was born. Up until that time I'd been breastfed and carried continuously by my attachment-parenting mum. And then she was gone. She stayed three nights in hospital having Tom and for the first time we were separate beings. My dad tried to dress me to take me to the hospital to meet my new brother, but he couldn't get my shoes on my feet. He described them as old person's feet, puffy and spilling over the edges. He tried and tried but couldn't get the shoes on and, realising how swollen my feet were, took me to the family doctor. 'She's distressed,' she told him. 'Her body is demonstrating her separation anxiety beautifully.'

It feels as though I'm having separation anxiety once more, this time as the result of separating from my sense of self. One symptom all my friends and I share is anxiety. I've never been anxious before but I begin to get pins and needles in my fingers, tiny electric almost-pains. My fingertips feel as if they are being pricked from the inside out, a thousand miniature needles. I am suddenly aware of a sparking and jabbing in my fingers and hands, an offbeat, semi-painful morse code. The pricking becomes numbness sometimes, a spreading deadness, and when I touch my face, either my hand, or my face, feels like it belongs to someone else, and the skin I'm in is unfamiliar.

My friends, meanwhile, are experiencing other, classic anxiety symptoms that I recognise from my nursing: they are shaky, dizzy, sweaty, have dry mouths, headaches, tummy aches, palpitations. The sharing of our strangeness helps. I feel less alone. It's as though we all have chicken pox and are comparing spot formations. Patterns of perimenopause symptoms become the tapestry of our conversation. We form a perimenopausal WhatsApp group, describing, on the whole, our symptoms:

Just let out a huge fart in Lidl. The cashier literally jumped. Anyone else farting all the time?

Back pain, joint pain, even my teeth hurt.

My eyelashes are shrinking.

I have a constant feeling of dread.

My eyes are so dry it's agony when I first wake up. Excruciating.

I have this weird metallic taste all day.

I thought I was having night sweats. But realised I have the wrong tog duvet.

Bleeding gums again.

Anyone else's tummy loudly rumbling all day? Regardless of food?

I'm having the classics: Hot flashes, irregular periods, wanting to stab my husband in his sleep.

Are you guys getting turkey necks? Double chin out of control.

Most of the time the WhatsApp chat is simply a place to let off steam and laugh or moan. We rarely have any advice to give each other, and we delight in taking the piss out of wellness. The idea that we get to choose to live a better life is a ridiculous, beautiful myth in our society. That illness and death can be avoided, or that we can eat our way out of depression or exercise our way towards good relationships. If we are simply perfect enough, then everything is possible. We are bombarded with images of women doing it all, having it all, so much so that I'm sure most of us feel constantly lacking. Sometimes my friends and I respond to this with humour: send funny photos in response to well-meaning influencers' recommendations. Emma downing a large packet of edamame beans (*edamame are a good way to regulate hormonal challenges*), Teniola with ten fags in her mouth (*time to quit for good*), me in gymwear on the sofa eating a cheeseburger (*moderate exercise and a healthy diet are the way forward*), Joy wearing a huge fake Father Christmas beard (*GP said she could give me my hope back. Also my libido back with testosterone but it might cause an increase in facial hair. Asked Sebastian if he wanted a sexless marriage or a bearded wife...*)

The group keeps us together as our external selves unravel. A thread of connection between women.

The WhatsApp group, and my friends, hold me together somehow, remind me that I'm not alone in this. But I feel alone. As a single woman and a single parent, I feel suddenly weighed down with responsibility to an extent that feels entirely new. My limbs feel heavier as I climb the stairs, leaden. I think about the shoulder pain experienced by the women of Japan, the primary symptom of their menopause. The reporting of symptoms changed after HRT was mass introduced in the country, and the menopause was medicalised. A self-fulfilling prophecy. Perhaps something easier to define. But shoulder pain feels to me like truth. A simple image to represent the true location of pain. 'You look like you have the weight of the world on your shoulders,' my mum tells me.

The GP had told me that the HRT patches might take a few weeks to kick in, but exactly twenty-four hours into having a patch on my abdomen and I am almost euphoric. Of course, I mean normal, but it feels euphoric after so many months (years?) of not feeling like myself. It is like climbing back into my old skin or meeting a friend I haven't seen for far too long, yet recognise immediately. I feel mildly high. As if I've micro-dosed with magic mushrooms, the world is suddenly techni-colour, and I wonder how long it was in black and white, distorted. I had a bad bout of flu when I was much younger and I think back to that pure joy of feeling back to normal. I feel the same peace now. How often we fail to appreciate our bodies when they are simply working. I take large breaths. I can breathe. I suddenly have energy. A simple thing, but the energy burst makes me realise how deficient I have been of both happiness and will. Everything took effort of gigantic proportions, even simple things like cooking dinner, making a bed, answering emails. Now, the house is eerily organised, my work up to date, and I beam with smiles when the children return from school.

'What's happened to you?' they ask me, suspicious, used to the zombie mum.

'I'm perimenopausal,' I tell them. I ask my daughter – who is fourteen – what perimenopause is. She shrugs. She's a bright, politically active and engaged young woman who is open about her body and not at all secretive about puberty. But she doesn't know what all women – including her – are likely to face in their forties.

'Menopause is when your periods stop,' she says, 'and you go a bit mad.'

I look at her for a long time. I wonder if this stigma and lack of understanding is some form of internalised misogyny, but whatever it is, I'm determined to talk honestly and openly about perimenopause with her, so that when it happens to her, it comes as less of a shock. I never want it to hit her as it did me, for her to suffer with it as I have. So I explain what perimenopause means. Or at least, as far as I understand it. My daughter looks horrified. My son covers his ears.

We have work to do.

I have work to do. I feel functional, able to cope better, sleep better. I can think properly. I might not need to move to the desert in Utah after all. Colours are brighter, food tastes better, music sounds clearer, poetry causes a beautiful ache in my chest. The last few months I have felt the opposite of that. Colours were dull, food tasteless, music annoying, and even poetry left me empty and hollow. It was as though I had fallen out of love with myself. I want to challenge that. I don't want to creep away from intensity. I know exactly what I must do.

I must put on the HRT patches. Keep going to therapy. And I must fall in love.

I think about my friends in relationships and our conversations about their changing bodies. How self-conscious they say they feel with their spouses about their bodies. Is this really a good time to share parts of myself, including my body, with another human? Yet I so desperately want to fall in love again. I keep remembering that time I felt my quilt on fire. The intensity of that moment, the feeling of being completely inside myself.

'I need to start dating again,' I tell Joy. 'Before my body gets even more out of control.'

'I have a friend of a friend that you would get on with,' says Joy. 'One of Sebastian's work friends.'

Blind dates, set-ups, are something to be avoided at all costs. The only times I've ever been on them have proved disastrous. Which is strange, considering friends should know you better than you do. But they've been among the worst dates I've ever been on, and I've spent the evening looking at the other person with a baffled expression, wondering if the matchmaking friend perhaps doesn't like me. Joy, though, I know, loves me and has known me since forever.

'He's really nice. Honestly. What have you got to lose? Not all straight men are dickheads.'

I'm nervous. I have anxiety dreams the night before, and my perimenopausal brain runs through every eventuality and possible disaster. By morning, my eyes are red from poor sleep and my skin is drier than it's ever looked. I can see the missing collagen. My face is at a weird half-way point between skeletal and puffy, with some sort of menopausal bloat. I'm a hybrid animal, chipmunk crossed with urban fox. I notice two grey eyebrow hairs and pluck them out, making my straggly eyebrows, overplucked in my teen years, even thinner and weirder looking. I go to different areas of the house, in different lights, with a hand mirror, examining my chin and upper lip for random black hairs. I then use half a bottle of moisturiser and oils and anything else I can find that might hydrate my skin. It's too late for eight glasses of water a day. My make-up routine has always been shameful and my teenage daughter can't be in the room when I'm doing it. She shakes her head at me in disgust, and lifts her head high, walking out as though I'm a massive disappointment. First I put concealer underneath my eyes, then rub it pretty much everywhere. Foundation brushes, sponges and techniques have passed me by. Instead, I rub it on my face as if it's soap, and I've never moved on from bronzer – some things in life are a constant. I do now have to make a tricky choice with mascara: I can either have seemingly no eyelashes at all, or a smooth-ish forehead. One or the other, not both. The moment I open my eyes wide enough to apply mascara my forehead crinkles up like a ridged potato crisp. Lipstick on perimenopausal dry cracked lips is a dangerous business, so I stick to neutral. And then there's the dressing. I am seduced by anything leopard print, 'fun' or high fashion and therefore have no sense of style. I am not one of those women of my age who wear linen in muted colours and layers, and expensive-looking jewellery. I love my gold-plated hoops too much. One thing has changed with my dress sense, though, and that is Spanx. I have fat in areas I didn't imagine you could. I've read about 'menobelly' but I've yet to read about 'menoback'. I have breasts at the back of my body as well as my front, I realise. I am all for body positivity and I love women, and men, with curves. But on my first date in forever I do not want four breasts. I squeeze myself into not one but two pairs of Spanx, knowing full well I am risking a yeast infection.

Wojtech and I meet early evening for a walk around Richmond Park, a chat and a take-away coffee. I drive there and park nearby. I'm feeling a bit nervous. Not butterflies, exactly; it's closer to nausea, to be honest. I have never liked first dates. Although I'm an extrovert, they make me clumsy and awkward. This nervousness seems to be increasing with age, which makes no sense to me. I never know what to wear or say, or how to act. I can often resort to self-deprecating humour, or sarcasm, even sometimes laughing uncontrollably in a bizarre way. Joy tells me to Just Be Myself, which is good advice, except I really don't know who myself is these days. Still, I'm an optimist. I long to meet someone to grow old with. My parents and grandparents had those lifelong marriages that were also friendships and I feel the lack of that in my life, despite it being a full one. I take a few breaths. *You never know.* It's a bright windy day and the park is full of people milling around, joggers, families with children. I see him leaning against a tree, holding two coffees. He's handsome. I am impressed. He has a nice face. His face in real life, if anything, is better than in his photograph. He doesn't recoil when he sees me approach: a good start. We say hi and begin to walk slowly into the green of the park, towards the deer. He seems relaxed and friendly. He tells me of his family in Ireland and Poland respectively, his sister who's a florist, and his puppy – a labrador named Ryan who he couldn't bring out as he has 'behaviour issues'. We laugh. I tell him about my love of old films and long slow walks, my failure to not burn cakes, and my political anger.

But thoughts keep splintering inside my head. My voice is normal and the chat is normal but I feel the real me bursting to get out, a perimenopausal Incredible Hulk. As we walk, I banish the anxiety going on in my head: *Lyme disease is caused by tick bites and deer have ticks and Lyme disease produces all the same symptoms as perimenopause and is hard to diagnose so you might die.* Out! Begone. Then, *You ate lentils at lunch and have a bloated stomach. He will think you are carrying twins, and assume IVF, that you're searching for a baby daddy.* Vanish! Get out! Or, *He might actually like you. Then you will need four more dates and you'll have to have sex with a perimenopausal vulva,* and, *I wonder if lubricant would stain my new Egyptian cotton duvet cover? It is White Company (sale) and costs a fortune (even on sale).* I push all these thoughts out of my head and manage, somehow, a nice, normal date with a seemingly nice, normal man. An hour in and he asks more personal questions. He begins coming across as fairly intense. Or maybe I am imagining it? Either way, the mood between us becomes awkward and a bit stilted. Dusk comes. I suggest it's been lovely to chat but I need to be getting home. We walk back towards the park exit, and towards the car, as the sky changes rapidly to night. He seems relaxed and chatty again, so I was probably just on high alert. Suspicious.

My car is parked awkwardly as ever and makes him laugh

out loud. I smile. We suggest another walk, another time. All is well. I've contained the weird anxiety and managed to not come across as too eccentric. We kiss on the cheek, and I walk away and turn back, awkwardly waving at a distance, then climb in the car. He waves goodbye. We have been chatting for hours. I didn't feel any fizzing chemistry, and we don't have much in common. But it was a nice time. A reminder. Whatever happens with this man, there are good men in the world. There is a world of dating that is actually OK. *Not all straight men are dickheads.*

But then, as I pull away and head down the road, I look in my rear-view mirror and Wojtech is chasing after me, shouting. I drive faster. He runs faster, shouts louder. He looks unhinged, his arms and legs flailing around. He's shouting and shouting.

I Love You.

I Love You.

In that moment, driving at speed, a memory: I am young. Twenty, maybe, in bed with a man I've been dating. We are having sex, I cannot call it making love, as he's just pummelling me from above as though kneading bread. He has a faraway look in his eyes and is screaming, 'Je t'aime! Je t'aime, je t'aime,' so loudly my flatmates bang on the wall. He doesn't stop, in fact gets louder. And he's not French. At all.

I put my foot down harder. Wojtech shouts again. Louder too. And then I hear him, clearly for the first time.

He is not shouting *I Love You*. He is shouting 'Your Lights. Turn on Your Lights.'

But by now I'm already crashing the car into a bush.

We don't have a second date. But I do learn many things from him. I learn that not all men love me, in either English or French. And I learn that along with everything else perimenopause is doing to my body, it also causes hearing loss.

4

Smell My Fingers: Dating

I am fourteen years old working Saturdays at the Market Café, where I clean ovens and try not to listen to my mean co-worker who barks orders at me as if she's a military commander: *Put some welly into it, girl; That's not a burn, you just have sensitive skin; you were late back from your break so I'm docking your wages.* It never occurs to me to consider her life, the fact that she is probably going through the menopause in this hot, stinking kitchen, and trying to manage me as a precocious teen refusing to remove the badge on my T shirt that reads: Fuck Off; I quote the Human Rights Act whenever she suggests I take it off. I didn't imagine being here, doing this. I doubt she did, either. The kitchen is heavy with grease and the smell of egg and bitter disappointment.

It's not my only job. I do a paper round until I get found out dumping papers in Dog Shit Alley, and a milk round, where I help the local milkman, in the dark early mornings that always seem to be winter. I learn to hold six freezing cold milk bottles between my fingers at a time, and my hands are permanently blue. I go from freezing to boiling, from ice-cold milk to burning hot ovens, as if I'm in a Swedish bath house. I babysit a boy who is completely blind and likes to play cars. 'Pass me the green car,' he says, and when I hand him the yellow car he holds it, running his thumb over it, then smells, and finally licks the car before he shakes his head. 'The green one.' And I spend a year or so thinking about whether colour has a shape, a smell. What does purple taste of? Even now I eat M&Ms with my eyes closed.

Make yourself useful and empty the ashtrays.

She sends me out of the kitchen to the main café area, to empty ashtrays into a large plastic tub. It's my favourite job, because if someone has left a decent butt I pocket it and collect ten or so to smoke the equivalent of a cigarette, after wiping the edges of spit and lipstick off with the washing-up cloth. Then there he is. A boy, maybe a year or two older. Green eyes, black hair. He watches me hold up a cigarette butt to the light, as if it's a rare gem. And he smiles. I notice he is wearing a shirt and a very thin tie, which I find wildly exciting. People round here only wear ties for funerals, or traffic court. I grab the small notepad, and promote myself. 'What can I get you?'

He has a book on his lap, which he lifts onto the table, face up: Nietzsche.

I picture our wedding.

'What would you recommend?'

I feel like a hostess in a fancy restaurant. I reel off the items least likely to give him salmonella. 'Avoid the omelette. And quiche.'

He orders a jacket potato and cheese.

I pile on so much cheese you can barely see the plate, and my 'senior supervisor' tells me I will put them out of business if I serve that much cheese on a potato. *We're not a charity, Christie.*

The plate is so cheese heavy I nearly drop it. But he eats it all. Quickly, like a wolf. I apply lipstick while he is eating. My boss looks from me to the boy, then rolls her eyes and smacks her forehead with the palm of her hand. I wait ten seconds then go to collect his plate. He writes his name on my arm in biro, Arron, and the words 'Sat 4' and his phone number. After he leaves, I take an emergency break and smoke all the cigarette butts without wiping the ends with a dishcloth. Even death can't touch me. I don't wash my arm all week; I'd have tattooed my arm if I could. It is the most romantic thing that could happen to me. I replay it over and over:

'Meet you outside Macdonald's on Saturday,' he had said, smiling, and I noticed he had a snaggle tooth, a chipped edge, and the following days I think about that tooth all the time. His thin tie, reading material and snaggle tooth all seem at odds with each other, which makes him even more deeply fascinating. I can still picture that snaggle tooth. I imagined my tongue against it, how sharp it would feel, if it would make me bleed.

I spend the rest of the week working out what I will wear. It needs to say casual and not too try-hard, while also naturally and effortlessly cool. I apply six layers of mascara, waiting between each layer for it to dry, until eventually my eyelids half close with the sheer weight. I look sleepy, which is good – nonchalant. The outfit is trickier. I want to look older than my fourteen years, naturally, but all my clothes seem suddenly very young. I curse Tammy Girl and the stall on the outdoor market where I buy fake Kickers and neon boob tubes and the entire NaffCo54 brand. I go for DMs, a checkered shirt, and baggy jeans with a chain hanging off them. I am in my Bros phase. I smother my skin in Superdrug self-tan, and spray more Sun In onto my dry orangey hair. I wear a thin black lace choker and remove the badge that says Fuck Off. I don't want to come across intimidating. Or intense.

I go first to my friend Natasha's house. Natasha is an expert at relationships, a love guru. She has been with the same boyfriend for four whole months and is on the pill. She takes the pill at school, during lunch, leaving the packet on the table like a dare to the teachers to mention anything. They ignore us. Then we go to the woods. The woods are where Natasha and I smoke Superking Extras, and put the world to rights, and where once during a cross-country race I sat and read for an hour, then took a taxi to the finish line. Natasha ignores the boys our age, who she says are immature losers. 'All except my Philip, of course. And Ben.' Bible Ben, as the mean kids call him, is a boy in another class, who is aloof and mature and wise, and can quote from the scriptures. We went to nursery together aged three and even then he seemed to know things about the universe. Natasha, though, is the real prophet. We queue up as she reads our palms, folding our hands into fists to check the lines at the sides, to tell us how many children we will have. *Half a line.* She gives me a poignant look. *Miscarriage. Or abortion.* We hang on her wise words. *Everyone else is a bell end. All the boys our age.* It is true that the boys our age seem particularly immature. They smell each other's fingers, to guess who they've been fingering, to prove they have. *Smell My Fingers. Scampi fries.* A thick layer of pheromones and Lynx Africa hangs over our lunchtimes in a thick mist.

The Stevenage clock tower looms over a small fountain near enough that I keep walking around the corner to check the time. These are pre-mobile phone days and watches are for old people. 3:55. I stand leaning against the Macdonald's window, wondering which side he'll be coming from, and what my best angle is. Time ticks on. 4:05. 4:10. By 4:20 I know in my bones he's had a terrible accident like Deborah Kerr's character in *An Affair to Remember*, and is likely unable to walk again, and we'll probably meet years from now, get married, and laugh together. 4:30. Maybe there is another Macdonald's in Stevenage? 4:40. What will I tell my friends? They will laugh at me. It will ruin my life. The most embarrassing thing to ever happen in the history of the world. Still, I am determined not to move. My teeth start chattering and it gets dark – it is March, and I don't have a coat. Nobody my age wears coats in winter in Stevenage. We are permanently mottled. But I can feel my feet freeze up in my DMs and my fingers begin to burn like I'm holding frozen milk bottles. I wait one and a half hours. Then walk home, crying my mascara off, until my eyelashes feel lighter.

I'm still crying on Monday morning. I ignore the bell at school and hang around the bin area until Ben walks past. He's earnest, never late. 'Where's Natasha,' I sob. 'My life is ruined.' He drops his bag and almost runs at me, pulls me towards him. His skin smells of Fanta.

'What happened?' His hand wipes the tears from my cheek.

I can't get my words out. He rubs my back until I can breathe. 'I got stood up,' I whisper. 'He didn't show. I waited an hour. And a half.'

He stops rubbing my back, takes a step backwards. 'Is that it? I thought something terrible had happened.'

I look at him. Despite the no-uniform policy that first attracted me to this school, Ben is wearing smart trousers, and his shoes are polished. I'm wearing a swimming costume under my T-Shirt and my Fuck Off badge. 'He just didn't turn up,' I continue. 'I stood there freezing for ages.'

Ben half-smiles, then sees me watching his face and shakes his head as though his smile is a drawing and his head is an Etch-a-Sketch. He picks up his bag. 'We're going to miss registration,' he says. But his eyes do not leave mine. I'm expecting him to say something profound and comforting, something biblical and wise. Instead, he looks confused. 'You just met him, right?'

I nod. 'Best person I ever met. I just know something *terrible* must have happened and I have no way of getting in touch with him ever. His phone number isn't working and I don't know where he lives. He's the love of my life. I know it.'

Ben glances away, at the school. He does not like being in trouble. He doesn't even like standing here, loitering near the bins, where kids make bin fires, or smoke hash. It's a miracle we're friends. 'Let's go in. You'll be OK.'

'You don't believe that can happen do you, but my uncle met my aunt when she was fourteen. It happens. Sometimes people who know each other forever, grow old together.' I start coughing. 'I need one of Natasha's Superking Extra cigarettes. I might as well die.'

I'm expecting Ben to tell me I'm too young to meet the love of my life. Or that we are going to be really late. Or that I shouldn't smoke Natasha's Superking Extra cigarettes, but he leans his arm on mine. And looks straight at my face. And he whispers. 'He doesn't deserve you.'

My other friends and I hang around parks, and drink Mad Dog 2020, and occasionally go 'night fishing' at Fairlands Valley Lakes, our parents never once questioning our lack of fishing equipment, or indeed fish. We lie around in tents drinking more Mad Dog 2020 and Get Off with each other, teenage bodies clasped together in sleeping bags, the one-man tents resembling near-term pregnant bellies punctuated with the outline of skinny limbs.

At fifteen I run away from home. I make it as far as my friend Sophie's shed. 'I'll live here,' I tell her. 'Until I can find something more permanent. Probably a flat in London.' She brings me some rolls that she's stolen from dinner. I graffiti on the shed wall: Christie 4 Arron 4 ever. But by evening time my mum has realised where I am and is sitting outside Sophie's house in our car – a blue, blocky Lada that makes a popping sound and belongs in the 1970s Soviet Union. Our car is so out of place in 1990s Stevenage that people literally stand and laugh at it, and I spend years telling my mum to *never ever pick me up from school*, or *park around the corner* and instead she parks right outside wherever I am and plays loud reggae with all the windows open. *You MORTIFY me*, I tell her. I can hear her pull up from where I'm sitting in the cold shed, and she begins honking the horn and shouting. 'I'm not leaving until you come out so you might as well hurry up.'

I go home sheepishly, my pockets full of stolen bread rolls, my mouth full of shame and rage. The next year I focus on playing the trumpet, and attending music school every weekend, and swimming for my county, as well as finding time to remain a peak teen, but I don't stop obsessing about Arron, about all boys. I spend an entire year with hair wet from swimming and lips red from playing the trumpet. I wear a swimming costume underneath my clothes every day, telling my mum it makes it quicker to change. Really, I just like the look of the straps. I am desperate for a serious relationship. For love. A lifelong best friend who I fancy too. But even with wet hair, which is considered a gold standard in the age of wet-look gel, and red lips despite the lipstick ban at school, and swimming costume straps, I can't get a real boyfriend.

I did not want to be single as a teen. And I did not expect to be single at midlife. My ex and I split after twelve years together. In the last few years of our relationship, we were both hanging on by our fingertips; neither of us, I suspect, wanting to face the prospect of being single despite us both knowing deep down that we were wrong for each other. The notion of doing life alone, especially as a single parent, was terrifying. So too now is the idea of dating, of getting back out there. The thought of being vulnerable, of being open with my heart.

After our split, I rent a small house for me and the children in Bromley. 'Bijou,' the estate agent says, which means it's small and a bit cramped. It's all I can afford, barely, and the kitchen and living room are basically the same room. There's no space for twelve years' worth of stuff, and I sell what I can, before giving some to charity, then hiring a skip for the rest. In our old house before we move out for good, I am surprised to find how unattached I am to the things that once felt so important. Knick-knacks collected over the years, ornaments, souvenirs from holidays. I look at my wardrobe, bursting with clothes of the person I was, that I thought I was, and I don't recognise them as mine. I tell my ex he can take whatever he likes of our kitchenware. I think of all the dinner parties I've thrown over the years; elaborate, stressful affairs involving too many courses, days of preparation, and hours of cleaning up. A fish poacher. A bread maker. Gifts we've received: an antique candlestick, a modern lamp, a picture of taxidermy butterflies, a stylish yet uncomfortable and broken Swedish antique sofa. Other furniture I upcycled, spending months, maybe years, scouring markets and sanding and painting ugly into beautiful. Old into young. I even went through a decoupage phase, and we have various lamps that I spent so much time on, and now realise look ridiculous. I thought I was an elaborate dinner party, upcycle, decoupage type of woman. I look at the brightly coloured butterflies, still and flat behind glass, perfectly symmetrical. I touch the Farrow and Ball painted walls, that I was so obsessed about, and smell the curtains I'd had made in our first year. They smell of another place. There's a large pot in the kitchen, too dirty and broken to go to the charity shop, beyond cleaning. I think of all the things it contained. The juniper-soaked Christmas ham I'd made for guests. The endless Sunday roast dinners. Goose fat potatoes. I think of Christmases and better times. Family times. There's a power washer in the garden, also broken, which I'd thrown in a fit of rage when I was pregnant, at the garden wall. I rest my head on the wall. Both the wall and my head feel cold and crunchy.

I spend money I don't have on removal men for the stuff I can't leave behind. The children and I sit on the floor of our new home, surrounded by brown boxes written on with Sharpie: Bedroom, Kitchen, Important. And we cry. The three of us sit and cry and cry, and look at each other as we do so, try and outcry each other. Then, we huddle together like penguins trying to keep out the icy cold. The removal men weave in and out and around us, not looking at our faces, not knowing what to say.

When my mum comes to stay shortly after we move, we eat breakfast on the second-hand sofa I found at The British Heart Foundation shop. It is not at all stylish, and extremely comfortable. There is no table. 'Where's your cereal?' my mum asks. 'You need to eat.'

It is true my skin is hanging off me like an old coat, my collarbones a coathanger. 'We only have three bowls,' I say. And when she looks horrified, 'We'll rotate.'

She puts her bowl down on the floor. 'We can go shopping today. You can't live like this.'

I try and smile. I am becoming expert at fake-smiling. 'The stuff you own ends up owning you,' I tell her. 'I read that somewhere.' I read a lot of things. My books survived the exodus. I stack them up against walls, and sometimes at night there is a bashing sound and I come down to find the floor covered in forgotten titles, and I sit amongst them and read until dawn. Inside these books I find comfort. There is solace in escapism, in time travel and poetry and stories. My physical friends save me during dark times, and my fictional friends do too. That I've always had trouble separating reality from fantasy, real from not, is not a curse after all, it is salvation.

'We can stock up,' my mum says, horrified at the way I now live. 'You can't live without stuff.' She picks her bowl up and rinses it, then dries it and starts filling it with cornflakes. 'You're not a student.'

Marina Benjamin, in *The Middlepause*, eloquently describes the self-destructive desires that are perhaps subconscious at midlife, but often unavoidable: 'in menopause a woman is forced to negotiate an entirely new psychic terrain, largely in the spirit of alienation. It is an eerie place, spring trapped with out-of-body experiences and veil-lifting moments that expose jarring, pop-up truths... suddenly you want to pack it all in, give up your job, blow up your marriage, leave the country.' Being single at this age may not be what I imagined, but I'm not alone in being so. As the years go by, friends around me start separating. Marriages fall apart. Relationships undone. I begin to see loose threads everywhere. There was a time in our late twenties and early thirties when almost every weekend was taken up with a wedding. And there is a time, a decade or more later, when every weekend is taken up with desperate, angry and confused friends who are sobbing on the phone about their relationship breaking down. 'The problems often pile up like a car crash,' Susie Orbach, psychotherapist, writes in an old article for the *Daily Mail* that my neighbour shows me. Orbach describes midlife: 'parents get ill and need round-the-clock care, teenagers full of attitude require constant emotional support, older children fly the nest and leave us wondering how on earth to fill the lonely evening hours. It's at this time, I've found, that marriages often falter and women begin to lose confidence in their sexual selves. Some find the decline of youth and beauty a source of grief and shock. Meanwhile, the menopause arrives, seeking out our vulnerabilities like a guided missile, just as we need all our strength to cope with daily life.'

I have an increasing number of single, middle-aged friends. We are like windswept pirates, rum drunk, wild-eyed, weather-beaten and cynical about life. We live lives of extremes, all or nothing. Lone parenting means a good proportion of our time is solely focused on family life, and a social life revolves around the children, or costly babysitters. But there are sometimes weekends without children at all, when they visit their dad, something not experienced by friends still in couples. The house is completely empty, lie-ins are possible, and friendships change in this space, mirror a child-free time of our lives.

Like many of my single-parent friends, Orla and I are dou-ble agents. After extended periods of sole-charge parenting, any rare, child-free weekend feels like being let out of a cage, a won-derful regression into aliases. We drink and dance until 4 a.m. as if we are twenty and on a girls' holiday in Ayia Napa, instead of in our mid-forties and fifties, in a quiet pub in Dulwich. The difference is the hangover. Joint pain. Dry eyes. Nowadays, my body screams at me if I drink any more than two glasses of wine or if I stand for too long, let alone dance all night.

'Remember when we used to go out all night then straight to work,' Orla says, groaning. We're lying in our dressing gowns, swiping away at Orla's dating app. We've eaten, for breakfast, a recreation of a pizza I once had in Sweden: 'Kebab

Pizza', basically an entire kebab's worth of meat, on top of a margarita pizza, smothered in garlic and chilli sauce. On the coffee table in front of us a giant bowl of chilli Doritos, two glasses of Berocca, a packet of paracetamol, another of ibruprofen, two Yakults, a pot of coffee.

Orla is recently back on dating apps, following the usual on-off pattern that most of my single friends and I adopt. We'll join an app, scroll relentlessly, go on a few horrific dates, then, emotionally scarred, come off the app and swear never to go back on again. A few months later we are back. This seems to be the modern-day drug of choice. Ultimate procrastination.

'Middle-aged dating is like a grotesque contact sport, with too many players, where nobody wins,' I say. 'A world where the focus is on beginnings rather than endings. A perpetual spring at the end of autumn.'

'Uh huh,' Orla doesn't look up. We're good enough friends that she doesn't need to put her phone down as I waffle on, and she scrolls as we chat, then occasionally holds it up, asking, say, 'what is it with men?' or, 'does this approach really work for him?' and then shows profiles, reflective of the heterosexual online dating world:

A man with a bandage around his head, lying in a hospital bed: *Dean. 56. Had a rough time recently. Looking for someone caring;* an extraordinary number of men holding large fish or next to live tigers; standing next to sports cars; giving Ted talks; or photographed with their children, and sometimes, wives; the polyamorous kink-friendly open-relationship sorts, who are often bearded and seemingly always bake bread; men bungee jumping off cliffs, or parachuting out of aeroplanes, or running across the Kalahari deserts; So. Many. Rock. Climbers; the afro-wigged men wearing novelty glasses, *having a Great Time, YOLO. My life is Awesome, I'd like someone to share these Good Times with;* the intellectuals; the 'naturists' who want to FaceTime; the feminists; the writers who will one day finish their bestselling manuscript; the newly divorced sad-eyed men who are clearly ten years older than their profile age suggests, and searching for someone twenty years younger; or, bizarrely to me, extremely young men, in their late twenties or even teens, looking for women twenty or thirty years older.

Menopause specialist Dr Louise Newson says that she can tell in a room full of twenty of so women who is receiving HRT and who isn't based on how happy they seem and the way their skin looks. I have one friend on HRT who, at forty-seven, is currently shagging her way through a Toy Boy Warehouse. She seems perfectly happy. With excellent skin.

I want to be happy, with glowing skin. After my disastrous blind date a few months ago, resulting in an almost car crash, I feel ready again to dip my toe in the dating pool. 'What should I say in my profile?' I hold my phone to Orla. My writing skills are useless when thinking about dating. I have no idea who I am, what I want, or certainly what I need.

I like books, films, jazz, walking and yoga. I'm looking for someone kind, who is interested and interesting.

Orla looks up. 'Best to be brutally honest.'

I tap in some words. Show her. We smile.

I'm hungover to fuck, in a dark room, currently watching back-to-back episodes of First Dates eating pizza and Doritos for breakfast. Shortly I have to take the car to the MOT centre in the industrial area of Orpington. Send help. And full-fat coke.

'Yup,' says Orla. 'Brutal honesty.'

We laugh, but we're not brutally honest. At all.

My profile picture is of me clean, wearing actual clothes, without a massive pizza belly, smiling and looking shiny. I look at my distended stomach post-kebab pizza and the chilli-sauce stain on my dressing gown. The room smells of meat. The windows and curtains are closed. The reality, and how I am presenting myself online, do not match in any sense. I can't remember the last time I washed my hair. I broke a hairbrush in it yesterday trying to brush it. I feel like we're living in a version of Sims, where we've created an avatar, and can give them the perfect life, from the comfort of my meat-smelling living room.

The first conversation, however, seems promising. I'm not very good at chitchat, I'm way too intense. I ignore Orla's advice to *keep it light and friendly*, to chat about films and books, or favourite foods, and instead I ask probing questions, as though I'm interviewing someone for a job.

'What's your relationship with your family like?'

'How was early childhood?'

'What do you think is your most annoying habit?'

Alex laughs at my probing questions. He has a normal-looking face and a normal-looking profile. No red flags. We text a bit, and he has banter and good chat, and makes me laugh. And we speak a few times on the phone. I am a bit nervous after my literal car-crash date, but after a few weeks of chatting, arrange to meet him anyway. We meet at Victoria station, after much discussion about where we should go. Alex has suggested a few restaurants and I've steered him towards the idea of a coffee or a drink, thinking that if we dislike each other it will be easier to leave, rather than be stuck together through an awkward meal. I am increasingly nervous. I've met people online before, of course, and had experiences ranging from normative to horrific, but despite my scepticism, this is how people date now. I have friends who found the loves of their lives on dating apps, and I know a number of happily married couples who originally met online. It might be, according to Orla, a *fucking jungle* out there, but it's how many people fall in love.

I get butterflies even now at my age, which strikes me as ridiculous. He arrives late but apologetic, and although a good three inches shorter than he had claimed on his profile, he is good looking with a friendly smile, and seems easy to talk to. Funny, even. His clothes aren't offensive (I once met up with a man wearing a bright red suit who told me his nickname was Santa). We have a drink, and chat. It is nice; I am enjoying myself. The butterflies disappear and I stop worrying about the coffee-only rule. We go for dinner, after all. The restaurant he suggests is fairly quiet and we order and laugh and drink wine. I like this man, I think, his open honesty and intellect. He tells me a bit about his life, the good bits, like he's a hologram or an Instagram page of himself. I'd be interested to know what his exes say about him. What mine say about me. But we keep it light.

It is true he talks a lot about himself, but I don't mind that. I like finding out about him. He orders more wine, and leans back in his chair, and chats as if we've known each other forever. He doesn't feel like a stranger.

But then Alex reaches into his rucksack and brings out a glass jar, the kind you might put cotton wool balls in. There are no cotton wool balls in this jar. Instead, there is a giant spider – a tarantula, alive, moving and very real. I yelp. He laughs and laughs. 'Oh, that's Roger,' he says, placing the spider next to his plate. 'He comes with me everywhere.'

Alex was bizarre but harmless, and I do have some nice dates. However, after a few months more of online dating I'm clocking up an array of horror stories. I write Maya Angelou's words on a Post-it note and stick it on my fridge: *When someone shows you who they are, believe it the first time.* Now that I've thrown myself into this world, I am consumed with longing for a stable relationship. I'm craving intimacy. And it feels further and further away from possibility. Maybe I'm just unlucky? There is a bear attack man, an incel, a woman who plays love songs on her acoustic guitar outside my window at 3 a.m. My judgement is off. Love, since the Quilt on Fire days, is my blind-spot, my Achilles heel, my area of disability. I have analysed this so much over the years – why I trust, even subconsciously choose, the wrong people for me. Or why they choose me. It feels as though it's speeding up. Damage seems to be a drug to me. Cat-nip. For a few months everyone I meet seems to be a cheat, liar, gaslighter, emotionally unavailable or avoidant, irresponsible, even criminal. The red flags that exist for other people are almost calling me over rather than waving me away. My friends act as gatekeepers, and for a while, Orla happens to be at the place I'm having dates at, says hi, maybe even stops for a drink. Then I'll get a text, via her rational brain: NO WAY ABORT. And despite not seeing the person she does, I'll politely decline a second date. Her radar for fuck-ups is profoundly more developed than mine. I'm losing heart, but she cheers me on.

'It's a game of numbers,' Orla reminds me. 'Eventually, after thousands, you might find someone who's OK.'

'Call me romantic,' I tell her, 'but I'm looking for more than OK.'

Amy Krouse Rosenthal died ten days after her essay 'You May Want to Marry My Husband' was published in the *New York Times*. When describing the love of her life, her beloved soulmate, she talks of the things you might see on a dating app: salt and pepper hair, 6ft, lawyer. But the love spills onto the page when she moves on from that into authenticity, friendship, deep and surface stuff that nobody is looking for but makes a person unique: 'Jason is compassionate–and can flip a pancake.' It is these details that contain the magic of him, of their relationship, of what she wants for him after she's gone: 'This is a man who, because he is always up early, surprises me every Sunday morning by making some kind of oddball smiley face out of items near the coffeepot: a spoon, a mug, a banana.' That she wrote these idiosyncrasies from her deathbed shows the importance of the mundane, how the ordinary can be the extraordinary. It seems to me that these unique small things are what make us who we are–not our height, build, job, ability to take a good selfie. The details of who we are and how we act form the heartbeat of a relationship. The rest is gravy. Amy's gift to Jason wasn't the permission for him to find love again. It was seeing him. Really seeing him. What psychotherapist Esther Perel calls true intimacy in her Mindvalley Talk, 'Balancing Love & Desire': *into-me-see*.

Helen Fisher, an anthropologist, suggests in *Why We Love* that dating is a game designed to 'impress and capture', which is not necessarily about honesty but novelty, excitement and even danger, which can boost dopamine levels in the brain. This feels timely. A chance for someone to see only the glossy, shiny version of you, and reflect it back. A chance for you too to see the glossy shiny version of someone else, until you don't. My idea of dating when I was fourteen and standing outside Macdonald's was certainly about impressing and capturing, and the last thing I wanted to reveal was my true authentic self. I wanted to be someone else, anyone else, a cooler, more sophisticated version of me. But now, in my forties, I crave authenticity, truth, being comfortable to be completely myself, warts and all. This yearning for realness is at great odds with the landscape of online dating. As I am quick to find out, dating is nowadays about many things. But it feels as if it is not at all about intimacy.

Perhaps we're collectively becoming good at lying, in this fake world of fake news and half-truths. Orla often texts me about potential matches. 'How should I respond?' And we make up an interesting scenario, a healthier, better, more luminous projection of her current situation. Instead of: 'I've just taken my screaming nephew to swimming lessons that he hates, and he vomited with rage,' we write, 'I'm listening to 6music, while making Thai food,' and instead of: 'I sent fourteen texts to my ex-husband last night, and now feeling a bit shit,' we write, 'I'm at a friend's book launch this evening in Mayfair.' 'I drank two bottles of Pinot Grigio at lunchtime and just woke up with my face in a bucket of KFC,' becomes, 'I'm interested in wine.' And: 'I just had a full-on row in the street with my neighbour who is a total prick,' morphs into 'I love living in London.' And 'I have listened to Madonna, the *Holiday* album on repeat for the last thirty years,' evolves into 'I love Wagner too.' My friends and I are lying our arses off.

We take a trip and decide to give ourselves fake names and jobs, and tell everyone in the bar we are part of a seal research unit. This would be juvenile even for teenagers but the fact that we are writers, and nurses, and lecturers, and middle-aged mothers, makes it even more ridiculous – but still, it seems, funny. We are staying at my mum's house in the Isle of Man, as we can't afford to go anywhere else but need a break, and she is away. She's left instructions and a card saying HAVE FUN with the words underlined. And then WATER THE PLANTS AND DON'T FORGET TO LOCK WINDOWS.

I am horrified that my mum would leave a note like this to an adult, almost middle-aged daughter, an academic professional. It is not how I imagined my life to be. I wonder if you start to believe the story you tell yourself, the lies, the projections. To protect myself from the truth. That I am in my forties, and despite having the illusion of being a professional, successful, independent woman, I'm stuffing my face with a bowl of chips, cheese and gravy, which I bought with the £10 that my mum left for me.

We go to see the seals the next day, at the Calf of Man, the bottom tip of the island, all of us dressed in thick winter coats, and shouting into the wind. We watch the seals intently as if we really are seal researchers. And tourists walk past us, watching us intently too to see who – or what – we are. We seem frightening, a gang of midlife unhinged wild women, shouting at the sea. We shout seal noises. And flap our hands against our sides as though mimicking seal body language. The people walking past say nothing but the seals respond and we shout back and forth a while, across the angry Irish sea. The seals have inky, glossy faces that disappear into the grey surf.

'Is anybody out there?' I continue. 'Can anyone hear me?' I listen for the seals but there is no response at all, and my voice simply carries off in the wind.

5

A Flash of Humanity: Sex

One of the most surprising side effects of HRT, for me, is the fact that is has turned me into a sex maniac. Well, not exactly, but I do suddenly start thinking about sex all the time. In France, the journalist Helena Frith Powell reports that women experience fewer negative symptoms from the menopause by having more sex, and the commonly held attitude is that this time is an opportunity to shake things up. The menopause is seen by many, positively, as a second adolescence. Adolescence for me was bad enough the first time. I am not sure I want to shake things up. I'm already over online dating. And yet I find myself thinking about sex every two seconds. I'm perplexed about this midlife sexual awakening, and more than a little disturbed by it. I start to wonder if other women are thinking about sex all day too, midlife women like me. I discover that I'm far from alone. In Louise Foxcroft's *Hot Flushes, Cold Science: A History of the Modern Menopause*, she describes a time in the late 1880s when 'some menopausal women came to physicians suffering from "pent up sexual longings", which were, they said much worse than mere pain: "no sooner does night come on I am prey to such dreadfully sinful desires that drive me mad". I had imagined sexual longing would just quietly creep away and I'd be left with other pursuits, like gardening. Instead, my body aches. My mind is an erotic playground. I can't seem to think of much else. I start to watch older women on the bus, at the shops, in the park. They are eye-smiling. Their faces dance with secrets. Maybe all older people think about sex more than I'd realised. Perhaps this is because sex is the opposite of feeling numb and invisible, and, alongside birth and illness, is the closest we get to an extreme physical experience. Yet at my age, it seems strange and wrong to be obsessing about sex so much. It's distracting, walking around with a burning body and head full of eroticism. And it doesn't feel at all liberating. I'm far too English; I'm no chic Parisienne. I feel full of thoughts and memories and shame and weirdness. But nursing has taught me that all people are strange. I begin to remember, reflect.

The man in front of me has a hoover attached to his penis. I'm a student nurse on a short placement in the Emergency Department and I'm trying to keep a straight face and not act shocked, and simply fill in the admission paperwork. But it's not easy. His wife is shouting, 'You stupid bastard,' while he explains that he fell on top of it and quite often does the house-work naked. I am so embarrassed. One of the things that scared me the most about nursing was the idea of washing men's genitals, and during my first placement on a medical ward I gave the most ineffective bed bath in the history of the universe. I soaked a cloth in a bucket of soapy water, reached my hand under the sheets of a patient and sort of patted him down a few times before retreating. But this is worse. My face is red and hot and I'm somewhere between trying not to nervously laugh and trying not to cry. I feel my neck mottling with rash. The Emergency Department staff are not embarrassed, or they're able to hide it very well. I am learning that sexual injury after misadventure is more common than you'd think. The nurses here have seen it all. 'Now then,' the nurse in charge walks into the cubicle and smiles at the man, and his wife, who is still muttering: *you stupid bastard*. She puts on not one, but two pairs of gloves, and opens a tube of KY Jelly, and turns to face the man. 'This might sting,' she says. And I see her wink over the man's head, at his wife.

'People insert all manner of things in their vulvas or rectums,' Joy tells me later, when I recount the story. 'Even their urethras, if you can believe it.'

We spend the evenings in our south London house-share swapping nursing stories, the landscape of nursing and nature of human beings incredibly shocking to us. But it's Joy's Emergency Department stories of sexual misadventure that open our eyes the widest.

'Of course, you get all the sex toys you'd expect, and the occasional small animal you'd think was an urban myth. But it's astonishing what people stick into each other: rolled-up newspapers, tweezers, shoehorns, a tool bag *with tools*, a baseball, shower heads, stones, glasses and bottles, barbed wire, fish, chopsticks.' She shakes her head.

I grimace. 'Human beings are so weird.'

'And the middle-aged,' Joy whispers, 'You'd not believe it, Christie. Things I've seen already, and I've only been there six months. Women and men in their fifties. *Our parents' age.*' She blows her cheeks out as if she's just been sick in her mouth. 'Gross.'

My own mouth drops open. It is so shocking to me, not the weirdness of people's sex lives, but the ages of patients presenting. 'Who even *thinks* of sex at that age? Let alone has the kind of sex that leads to a trip to the ED?'

She laughs. 'I'm telling you. Nothing shocks me any more. Middle-aged people are having more sex than people our age. And they're massive perverts.'

This feels *tragic* to me at nineteen, Joy at twenty-three. Astonishing. Unbelievable. I am continually shocked throughout my nurse training, about mature people's sex lives. I am a bit prudish. But the patients and people I look after are most definitely not. And they are so incredibly, impossibly old.

*

I work part-time in a care home (which at that time we cruelly call 'old people's home' as if it's a knackers' yard for old horses) while I'm a student nurse and take extra shifts as a healthcare assistant too. I'm hoping to gain some sort of clinical knowledge but I also need the cash. The work in the care home is physically heavy and emotionally important. Dignity feels like a gift that is really difficult to wrap. Slippery. The residents are all – to me – ancient, and so close to death that they can barely move, between worlds. They sit watching TV in a day room, almost catatonic, and it feels pretty depressing and lonely, this reality of old age. Still, the care-home staff try to cheer things up, organising bingo, quiz nights, an early version of Zumba, which ends badly with a resident falling over and twisting her ankle. I remember her clearly, Edith. She is accident-prone but always pushing herself to join in everything. She's forever asking me to take her out for the day, 'to the seaside', and we do get outside whenever the weather is nice, but she is unsteady on her feet and so we encourage her often to use a wheelchair or a walking frame. She refuses. We watch her, unnoticed, in the background, from strategically placed points in the room, as if she's the president and we care assistants are secret service, lest she begins to wobble or get shakier. I love Edith. She wears leopard-print slippers and bright red lipstick, and a hand-knitted mint green cardigan you might see on a newborn baby. Her eyes are sharp and blue and she has a thick mop of fresh snow-white hair. She never eats the meals served up as she says they are 'dogshit' and instead has a Jammy Dodger biscuit in her hand at all times. She approaches every single day as if it is her last, with enthusiasm and a complete lack of fear, and I imagine that must be how she's always lived. She is ninety-four. A life well lived. Most of the other residents, I suspect, find her annoying, though. Despite everyone's efforts there is not a collective mood of cheerfulness in this place, but one of melancholy. The air is heavy. Many people in the care home are suffering, physically as well as emotionally. People are in pain, and many of them seem to be giving up, just waiting to die, one foot out of the door already. But a couple of the residents perk up when Edith makes an appearance, and it is wonderful to see Frank and Gareth laughing with Edith at lunchtime, them both eating the cottage pie while Edith munches her Jammy Dodgers. Both are quiet men in their late nineties who have mobility issues and a heap of co-morbidities that leave them fairly reliant on care-home staff for their daily needs. I haven't heard them laugh like that in a long time. And later, when we do 'pub quiz night', the trio forms a team, and they win.

It's a quiet evening, and there are only three of us on duty. The other two carers are changing the bed of a resident who is incontinent. I am dishing out the evening cups of tea. I knock on Edith's door. No answer. And it's locked. When you work with the very elderly, you worry when this happens. Deaths here are frequent, as are accidents of all sorts. My heart knocks in time with my fist. Edith is very old and frail. She seems more wobbly than normal and falling over a lot. Anything can and does happen. Dreadful images wait behind my eyelids every time I blink: of falls and cuts and injuries and head wounds and blocked airways, anaphylactic reactions, and in my ears I hear Kussmaul Breathing: a death rattle. Not Edith. Not yet. I try the door again, and shout for my colleagues. But they shout back that they can't come just now: *Code Brown*.

I try the door again. 'Edith, it's Christie. Are you OK?'

I am praying that she has not died. I love Edith, but also have not yet seen a dead body and I am afraid. I push the door, lean on it, and then finally, it opens.

Edith is not dead.

In fact, she is semi-naked in bed, along with Frank. And Gareth.

The realisation that older people do not suddenly stop having a sex life as they age is a complete revelation to me. That even *extremely old* people sometimes have sex. There are no older people talking about sex on television or in films, no talk of it in print media, or even in a social context. Lynne Segal, a Professor of Psychology and Gender Studies, wrote in the *Guardian*, that 'while signs of physical ageing are routinely played down in leading actors, who regularly take roles as still vigorous and desirable characters (whether heroes or villains), the opposite applies to older actresses, if they are allowed to appear on screen at all.' We are presented with the idea time and time again that sex belongs to young bodies. Sex resides in the Kingdom of the Well, and in the Kingdom of the Young. In many ways, there is nothing less sexy than ageing. Vaginal dryness, atrophy, prolapse, loss of elasticity or pelvic floor muscles, delicate skin that is easy to injure, increased pain, decreased blood flow, and the factors of tiredness, depression and insomnia, low self-confidence. Many women are suffering – with painful sex, tearing and ripping, soreness, inability to reach or difficulty having orgasm, itchy vulvas, weak bladders and incontinence. Yet, despite these symptoms, there is something raw in the fault lines, something wilder and more mysterious. There is beauty in the falling apart, a less polished, more honest version of expression.

During my thirties and now into my forties, I find I'm increasingly fearless, experimental and, at times, even selfish. Am I becoming animalistic, wild, even violent? With each year, I lose myself more in sex, fall into the spaces between reality and fantasy, climb totally inside my body and feel every electric cell. Of course, not everyone feels this way. I know plenty of women and men who have no interest in sex and are content, even happy, to be free of it at midlife, or at any age. But the idea of sex has become more important to me, and more sensory: I want to taste and smell as much as touch. I have the confidence of complete embodiment, inhabiting my shadows and dark places, without fear, until everything is more raw and vital. Different. As I turn towards the next half of my life where mortality is so much closer, I crave this. Sex has become more spiritual. It feels sacred: a deeper connection to another soul, but also my own. This is not a new notion. For Freud, religion was always about sex, while for Jung, sex was always about religion. Jung defined the libido as the totality of psychic energy, not limited to sexual desire. Perhaps my increasing libido and totally immersive sense of sexual self is reflective of a thirst for psychic energy, or religious understanding. Or maybe it's about identity and belonging, a way to know myself and others on a deeper level, naked in every sense, stripped of clothes and masks and niceties. Along with the challenges and changes of perimenopause, there is also a midlife of possibilities. Sex in my youth was simple pleasure, yearning and lust. At midlife, I am finding that it is vulnerability, truth, openness to intimacy. Sex means I can connect with another human being in a profound way and this thirst and hunger for connection circulates inside me, primal and powerful. *Le petit mort*, a flicker of something intensely and uniquely human. Two people seeing inside each other, for a hot minute. Midlife sex is a flash of humanity. But it's not for the squeamish.

*

I am bleeding in biblical ways. I had imagined menopause is about the cessation of periods, I'd perceived that they would get less and less, smaller and smaller until they vanish. My blood is shocking. The GP suggested that HRT, along with the Mirena coil I now have, might settle things down, and make my periods lighter, but nothing improves. Instead, I have never, ever experienced such heavy, long and unpredictable bleeding. One month I'm bleeding so heavily that I have to change a giant tampon every ten minutes, and in the end I give up and sit on the toilet, dripping blood out, every now and then doubling-over abdominal pains and a clot plops into the cistern, the size of a walnut. I have to wear a giant tampon and two sanitary towels and still, blood spills out of the sides and stains my knickers, jeans and once, on Alastair's sofa.

I meet Alastair at the train station. He's reading a newspaper and wearing nice shoes. He reads loudly, rustling the newspaper open large in front of him, turning the pages almost aggressively. I sit next to him and drink a coffee, and as he turns a fresh page he knocks my arm, and the coffee spills a little, onto my sleeve.

'Oh, I'm sorry.'

'Don't worry,' I say, rubbing the sleeve, and moving over.

'Delayed?' he asks. He has nice teeth, I notice. I like his red hair and short beard, a perfect auburn. He is wearing glasses, and as he nods his head at the board flashing with delayed trains they fall slightly down the bridge of his nose and he pushes them back.

I nod. 'Good excuse to sit and relax.'

He grimaces. 'I need to be in Oxford for a meeting an hour ago.'

He has a Scottish accent. He looks at me. he is wearing a suit so well ironed the creases look sharp. His eyes move a fraction over me. I'm wearing jeans and a hoodie and my trainers are dirty. This doesn't seem to deter him. 'I'm Alastair,' he folds the paper, carefully, until it too looks ironed.

'Christie,' I shake his hand. 'Anything exciting happening in the world?' I gesture to the folded-up paper.

But he doesn't look down at it. Instead, he looks right at me, and smiles. 'Maybe.' And he hands me a business card.

My train rattles into the station, and I consider missing it, but I'm already late. I smile, nod at his paper, 'enjoy the forced relaxation,' I say.

He looks from the train to me, as if trying to decide something, then shrugs. 'See ya, kid.'

I look at the card and try and ascertain if the quality of the paper is too curated, too *American Psycho*. I am also not sure if calling a grown woman 'kid' is endearing, or creepy, but in any case, I watch him as my train pulls away. And he watches me back.

Now, a few months of dating later, and it's me bringing the

horror: I'm bleeding so heavily I swear I can smell blood. Alastair tells me it's fine though there is terror in his eyes as he scrubs the sofa stain, then washes his hands for a long time, like Lady Macbeth. Out, damned spot.

'I'm not sure any of this is normal,' he says. 'That you *still* have a period?' he asks. 'I'm worried about it.' He shakes his head. 'It's not normal.'

And I start to worry too. I'm not normal, in any sense.

Another few months and another never-ending debilitating period. I visit the GP four times, convinced that it is cancer. Around the age of seventeen I had irregular and abnormal bleeding. 'You are too young for a smear test,' I was repeatedly advised. Times have moved on since then, and all GPs know that, although rare for younger women, cervical cancer can happen at any age. But by the time I had a smear test, I'd developed grade three pre-cancerous cells and needed treatment that was both painful and traumatic. It is twenty-seven years since then, but I can still smell my cervix as the doctor tried to burn off pre-cancerous cells. A mixture of burnt toast, and something sweet that is turning bad – like out-of-date apple sauce.

The GP tells me it is likely to be perimenopause and that some women can experience significant changes to their periods, but she sends me for investigations to be on the safe side. I have a smear test, a colposcopy and am sent for a transvaginal scan. 'I had an orgasm once during a transvaginal scan,' Orla later tells me. I am lucky. My scan is clear of cancer. They do discover adenomyosis, a condition that causes heavy bleeding, but it is not considered serious in my case.

Regardless, I find myself googling health conditions with increasing frequency and learn that prolonged or irregular bleeding *can* be a sign of impending menopause, but also some cancers, and even chlamydia. My tests come back clear, and I become convinced that Alastair has given me chlamydia, despite our carefulness. I have never had a sexually transmitted disease before, but there we have it, my time has clearly come. I tell him the outcome of my extensive Google research and he takes time off from his job to get to a sexual health clinic, only to report back that no, it is not chlamydia. He sighs, avoids my eye contact. 'I told you.'

I begin to cry. 'I don't know what's wrong with me,' I tell him. 'I'm paranoid, and anxious all the time.'

Alastair reaches out and pulls me towards him, and I snot cry onto his shirt. He moves slightly away, and kisses my head, reaching for a tissue. But instead of giving me the tissue, he uses it to wipe the tears and snot from his arm, looks at me, and tilts his head to the side. 'Maybe you're having a midlife crisis?'

Canadian psychoanalyst Elliott Jaques coined the term midlife crisis. In his paper 'Death and the midlife crisis', he described

'The compulsive attempts, in many men and women reaching middle age, to remain young, the hypochondriacal concern over health and appearance, the emergence of sexual promiscuity in order to prove youth and potency, the hollowness and lack of genuine enjoyment of life, and the frequency of religious concern, are familiar patterns. They are attempts at a race against time.'

Sexual promiscuity feels like hard work, but it's true I'm at the gym a lot. Joy and I are talking in the Pilates queue about *Love Island* and reminiscing about her nursing in the Emergency Department. 'It's just so manufactured,' she says. 'So unsexy.'

I get what she means.

'They should make a *Love Island* for the middle-aged. Send a bunch of the newly divorced to an island with a box of drugs and a few crates of Pinot Grigio. That's a show I'd watch. Much wilder and more interesting.'

It's a surprising fact that many of my friends are wild and fascinating and appear to be sexually liberated. Despite a mainstream narrative that sexual libido diminishes with age, midlife appears to be a time of sexual revolution for many people. But not all; there is, in my friendship group, also a clear split. I know women who have gone off sex entirely at midlife, and others who are becoming increasingly sexual beings. This can't simply be about menopause or physicality or bodies, as the divide is marked by those women who are married and in long-term relationships, and those who are suddenly single and suddenly hyper-sexual. Perhaps the peri-menopause is the switch itself, and it's all the other crap – life experiences, residual trauma, quality of relationships – that determines the direction of things, whether the light is switched on or off. An older school mum struggled with sex and libido for years. She kept telling me about her lack of inter-est, as if that part of her had fallen off a cliff, and she didn't think she wanted a sexual life any more. 'We haven't had sex in five years.' Now, after a brutal divorce she finds herself single and everything has changed. Everything. The expression on her face has altered, her eyes are different. She describes being full of desire and longing. She begins to hook up with men and women regularly, as if sex is a new hobby. She turns up at the school gate flushed and tipsy. She says she is drunk with sex, not alcohol, as she's spent the day shagging. She laughs all the time, and we watch her with intrigue and more than a little jealousy in her sense of freedom. The fact that she had no interest at all in sex with her husband and is now, seemingly, only interested in sex, suggests to me that this is not, for her at least, purely about a hormone deficiency. Sexual freedom at or after menopause is a culturally complex phe-nomenon. In Costa Rica there has been an increase in the incidence of human papillomavirus infections in menopausal women, reportedly due, in part, to more sexual freedom after menopause. For many women, in many countries, the end of fertility is the beginning of liberation.

Of course, hormone deficiency and the myriad perimenopausal symptoms play a huge part, and for some people sex is the first major casualty of midlife. My friend Sarah has not had sex with her husband in ages. After losing her libido entirely Sarah has seen GP after GP and been put onto antidepressants as her blood tests are normal. I have discovered that hormones fluctuate day by day, hour by hour, so are pretty meaningless at diagnosing perimenopause. But even after the antidepressants don't seem to be working, and the dose is increased, a second added, she is not offered HRT. 'Breast cancer in my family,' she says. Which is not necessarily a valid reason, though one that she's been told. HRT is not for everyone. One in ten perimenopausal and menopausal women in the UK are taking HRT, but that leaves nine out of ten managing without oestrogen, like Sarah. I wonder how on earth they do it. How they function at work and sleep, how they manage the responsibilities of midlife, let alone even think about sex.

'We're at breaking point,' Sarah tells me as we sit on a park bench watching the world go by: young mums pushing buggies, dog walkers, weed smokers, groups of laughing teens. 'I have absolutely no interest whatsoever. It's wrecking our marriage.'

That Sarah is uninterested in sex is especially surprising to me.

A mere few years ago. We are at a party in Cheshire, with friends who have recently moved there, and we are all in a Jacuzzi. Teniola's new friends are rich. There is a swimming pool, Jacuzzi, and even a changing room in their manicured garden. We are drinking champagne in the warm, bubbling water. Sarah puts down her glass and leans over to start kissing Emma, much to everyone's surprise, including Emma. Sarah stops and sits back, looks around at all the shocked faces; she looks surprised and confused. 'We're having an orgy, right?' She is bewildered that we are in a Jacuzzi without the possibility of an orgy. Teniola's new friends are horrified and quickly get out of the water as if it is full of jellyfish. Sarah, Teniola, Emma and I remain in the water, laughing and wondering if we are the strange ones, or they are.

'I don't think it's that sort of party,' I laugh. Sarah looks embarrassed. 'Don't ever change,' I tell her.

'I can't change,' she says, 'that's the problem. I thought I'd be a grown-up by now. I'm middle-aged and behaving like I'm a teenager.'

Alastair and I have been dating a few months, and this makes me feel like a grown-up. We go out for dinner, or to the theatre, or to jazz bars, where he nods his head in time with the music.

He's polite, old-fashioned, always walking on the outside of the pavement and opening doors. It is true that we don't talk much, and the long silences between us, when there is no jazz, feel vast at times, so I find myself searching for conversation. I ask him questions, and he talks about his work as a property developer, about the price of property, and I try not to zone out. He drinks expensive whisky and spends hours explaining the vintage of a single malt and despite hating whisky, I listen and try to learn. When I was a child my dad went through a stint as a wine buyer, and he'd tell me stories of the people and the soil, paint a portrait of place and time, until I could smell the narrative inside the wine, imagine it living and breathing, until I could taste the landscape it was grown in. He could read wine like books, as though each bottle was pure poetry: *heady, gold, hazelnut; honeysuckle butter; look at the tears dropping down, trying to reach the earth once more.* Of course, my dad made a lot of stuff up. And maybe I have daddy issues. Still, Alastair has no poetry for whisky. He kisses me hard with fiery, scratchy lips, then tells me how much the whisky cost. 'Forty-year-old blended Scotch. Eight hundred and fifty pounds.'

Alastair likes to talk about money. And he likes buying me gifts. He is generous. So when he presents me with a small bag of Agent Provocateur underwear I don't want to appear ungrateful. I try it all on and look at myself in the bathroom mirror. I look a bit ridiculous. And I can't get comfortable. We go out for a black tie dinner with some of his university friends from St Andrews. I am unable to sit still. I'm suddenly *aware* of my vulva. It's a part of my body that I hadn't really paid too much attention to, outside of the bedroom, and yet now it is demanding attention, itching, uncomfortable, throbbing in my knickers. It feels hotter than the rest of me too, as though it's taking on a life of its own. I can't get comfy in my seat. Despite me knowing that perimenopause sometimes causes vaginal atrophy, mine feels inflamed, angry, fragile and *swollen*. Which doesn't make me feel particularly sexy, despite the new underwear, which is infinitely sexier, I understand, than my Marks & Spencer staples.

I lean across to Alastair, and whisper. 'I need to take my knickers off.'

His eyes open wide and he licks his lips, nods enthusiastically. 'Yes, you do.'

'No, you don't understand. My vulva feels like it's swelling up or something. It's perimenopause I think. . .'

Alastair looks confused, cups his ear. The table is buzzing with conversation, his friends, all like him, are also drinking whisky and talking loudly. I suddenly feel very alone, and out of place. And I feel unsure if I like these people. Unsure why I am here, or who I am.

Alastair looks confused, he puts his hand on my leg. Grins.

I try leaning closer, speaking a bit louder. The restaurant is packed, and loud and people are drunk shouting. Nobody is looking at us or paying any attention so I try again. 'I need to take the underwear off. The knickers. I mean they're lovely and I really appreciate the gift. You're very kind.'

'What are you talking about?' Alastair says. He can't hear me.

I continue, slightly louder. Suddenly there is a lull in the conversation, a moment of quiet, a split second of silence above the din. And in that moment my voice shouts out:

'My vagina is the size of Brazil.'

Later Alastair stays over at mine, and we laugh about the incident. 'Don't worry,' he keeps saying, 'don't worry, nobody heard.'

I have somehow managed to keep the Agent Provocateur underwear on, and this pleases him. 'You look very sexy,' he says.

I don't feel sexy. The Mirena coil has, at last, helped the heavy bleeding, but my periods remain erratic. The never-ending perimenopausal period. I take out the giant tampon and put down a towel. It's a bit damp but I hope he won't notice.

I find some lubricant that I ordered online at the back of my cupboard, only to discover as I open it that it's candyfloss flavoured. I hold the tube of lubricant as if it's a relay torch. 'Candyfloss.' I wave the lube at him. 'We probably won't need it as blood's a pretty good lubricant, luckily.' I laugh.

He is quiet. But then laughs too. 'Not everyone is a nurse, you know.'

I imagine lovemaking and romance and that connection of

deep feelings towards each other. Instead, it's like a scene from *Jaws*.

The blood and candyfloss lube mix together and fizz like a chemistry experiment gone wrong. The room stinks of candyfloss and we are splattered with blood, our lower halves look like a Jackson Pollock painting. My Spotify playlist on shuffle picks out a heavy drum and bass tune.

He stops moving. 'I can't do this,' he says. He sits up. 'I'm fifty years old.'

It's all a bit too messy for him, I can see immediately. I'm too messy. Too real life. Too confronting. My honesty. I am full of rage and blood and lust and chlamydia anxiety. I open my mouth and all words and thoughts and feelings spill out, unfiltered. He holds my arms and my gaze as though he is trying to contain me, and yet I'm uncontainable. It will not work between us, I can see already. And if it does, I will have to shrink down and inwards, have to make myself fit the smallness of his perception of me, his want for an idea of me, not the real version. His want for an idea of him, not the real version. Midlife, for all its mess, its blood and gore, and confusion and madness, will not allow me that. Midlife is brutal honesty.

Sex with Alastair is not good. It makes me feel wrong, abnormal and embarrassed. We shower and get dressed and I make some tea, and we sit in my kitchen. 'I don't think this is working,' I say, 'I mean our sex life is terrible.' He looks so relieved. His body folds as he exhales.

'It's all a bit messy,' he says.

I smile, and he smiles too and the smiling between us feels honest and intimate. As though we see each other for the first time, and this part is the naked.

'I actually like the messiness of it,' I tell him. 'I think I need to find a partner who embraces that. And comfy Marks & Spencer underwear.'

He laughs.

This messy magic of being human.

6

Small Sharks: Wisdom

I'm underwater in a vast tank, unable to breathe, not even trying to. There is a window of glass, and I realise I'm in some kind of an aquarium. The blue-green water is ice-cold though my skin is numb. Or is it even my skin? I don't know, can't feel it. Everything is too blank, too cold. There are sharks circling, and water snakes, and an octopus is below me, its legs snaking around my ankles. The fish are sharp-toothed and move in shoals, making sinister, inky patterns in the dark blue. On the other side of the glass, people. They watch me, with unblinking eyes, staring at me, or rather through me. I am not human here.

This is a time of intense dreaming. I regularly wake to vivid and bizarre dreams, often nightmares. I bring my dreams to therapy. I tell Luisa about the dream I keep having about being in a giant tank, with fish and stingrays and sharks of all shapes and sizes. I am underwater and afraid, looking through the glass at a room that is much like the room we have therapy in. You don't have to be Freud to work out the basics. But Luisa is interested in what the sea creatures represent. 'You have things going on in your unconscious that your conscious brain hasn't or can't process yet. But therapy can help that. Dreams can speed up what it is we need to get at.' We work out together that the sea creatures represent romantic relationships, mostly with men that I have dated. The people I assumed I fell in love with. Where my quilt most definitely caught fire. When describing the character of some of the men in my life Luisa returns to the shark tank. We talk about my past relationships. The men I met online – a man who said he lives with his wife but they are 'clearly not together'.

'Did he say separated?' Luisa asks. Did he? I think he did. Maybe. But I'm learning that what I hear and what is being said do not always match up. But he definitely said they are not together. 'Shark,' she says. Another man who told me he would never live with another person. Another who talked of feminism and women's rights, and who I discovered had been frequenting brothels. Alastair, who showered me with expensive gifts yet seemed to switch off when I spoke. 'Shark,' says Luisa. 'Shark, shark, shark.'

What is more interesting, perhaps to both of us, is not my inability to spot sharks, but my inability to recognise seahorses, or starfish, or other, nicer creatures: whales, dolphins. 'There are all kinds of creatures in an aquarium, and they are not all dangerous.' Nice guys could be waving a flag in front of my nose and jumping up and down and I barely notice them. That is not to say I haven't met and had love affairs with healthy, kind and good people. I have had significant relationships with wonderful people that I will never regret despite it not working out. But now I'm in a dating tank, and it's impossible to work out which type of sea creature is in front of me.

'He seemed really lovely,' I tell Luisa more about Alastair. 'Nice. But I got a real sense he was a bit gaslighty. Quick to anger. He always made me feel a bit ashamed. Made me feel bad about myself. I mean that's not his problem, it's mine, I was too messy for him.'

She frowns. Then presses her mouth closed.

'He was a small shark, maybe?'

There's silence a moment, and then she laughs, a tiny bit. 'Perhaps it's best to avoid all sharks,' she says. 'Even the small ones. Especially the small ones.' Her eyes fill up with something of her own.

I'm not alone in this dating shark tank. 'He was waiting at the tube station with a carrier bag,' says Orla. 'I mean it wasn't even a bag for life! If he'd been carrying a bag for life on the date, I'd have met up with him again.' Success is relative. She goes on another date with a man, and a second date turns into a third. He offers to cook for her in his flat. And she phones up excited. Twenty years ago I remember her phoning me with this level of excitement. Her then boyfriend had proposed. She sounded so happy then and again now, yet the barometer of expectation has been reset.

'He had actual lampshades on his ceiling lights. No bare bulbs! I can't believe it. Actual lampshades...'

Our dating bar is so low that no naked light bulbs in a man's flat is representative of a male unicorn. Still, we plod on. We form another WhatsApp Group: this time, one for dating anecdotes.

Turns out he is a hoarder, and lives with his mum.

He called me after four months to say I should get checked out. He didn't even remember we'd used a condom.

He had ketchup – or blood – in his beard.

We went back to his for a glass of wine and he started talking about his ex-wife, then cried all evening.

He turned up at my workplace with donuts for my colleagues. We had only been on one date.

It was going so well until he took his top off. He had Jesus Loves Me tattooed on his chest.

Dirty penis.

My daughter's headteacher is on Tinder doing one of those top-off bathroom selfies.

Found some treatment for pubic lice next to his bed.

I go on this date with a poet who has holes in his trainers. He offered to give me a lift home. And when we walked over to the road there was no car there, instead a push bike. I was still baffled, but he took the lock off and pointed to the handlebars, 'you can sit on the front.'

Joy and I are dancing on a sticky floor to music that is blaring out so loud you can feel it in your chest. I have dragged her out, determined to enjoy the real world, and forget about dating and men. My feet hurt despite wearing trainers, and I've an early start tomorrow, but I refuse not to have fun. I remember our nights out in years gone by, how we are always the last ones standing, how Joy knows every word to every song. She's not singing now. 'Shall we get the bus home and have tea and toast?' she shouts. 'I'm knackered.'

I shake my head, vigorously, despite being knackered too. 'No way, we're here to have fun. Besides, I can't even eat fucking bread any more.'

The other people dancing look as if they too are forcing fun. Aggressive fun. There's a chair next to the DJ booth and I look at it longingly. But I refuse to give in to middle age. A man dances over, says hi, introduces himself: Clive. It's late now, and Joy is bored and tired. 'Let's go back and have Marmite on toast,' she whispers. Marmite is our drug of choice. I chat a short while with Clive. He's not particularly attractive but I'd have probably stayed and had a drink with him had Joy not been so desperate to go.

'Maybe we can get coffee sometime,' he suggests.

I'm not interested in dating and breaking up with Alastair is fresh and still a bit painful. I keep wondering if there's something wrong with me. It's nice, reassuring even, to get some attention. I put my number into his phone. No harm in coffee. I hand him the phone, and he winks, slowly, and I realise my error. He is not wanting coffee. I immediately regret handing out my number to a random man. But I don't think much of it. I'll ignore his calls.

Joy and I are home and in our fluffy dressing gowns drinking tea and eating toast within an hour. We both put slippers on. 'This is what it's come to,' I say, eating bread, after all.

In the days that follow I am surprised and a little relieved that Clive does not text or call. 'That guy was a bit weird,' Joy confirms. 'I can't believe you gave him your number.'

'I know. I don't know what's going on in my head these days. Maybe it was just a rebound flirt? Anyway, I'm glad he didn't text, to be honest.'

But he did text. Just not me.

Alastair calls me, angry. He is shouting down the phone. I can't make sense of his words, something about a dick pic. And

I think he must have lost his mind. His anger is palpable. The phone shakes with it. I see a flash of who he really is, always was, and I'm about to hang up. But then he says: Clive. And I realise what I've done.

It wasn't my number I gave to some random guy on that night out. It was Alastair's. Clive sent him a dick pic.

'I feel like such a failure,' I tell Luisa, after recounting this, and other disasters. 'I've failed at love.'

'There are many different kinds of love,' Luisa tells me. 'To say you've failed at love simply isn't true. Love isn't all about pragma.'

I like it when she speaks like this. She is wiser and older and teaches me more in an hour that I've ever read in books. 'What is pragma?'

She looks shocked. But her poker face returns, and we talk about love in all its forms, the enduring love that is pragma but also eros, ludus, agape, philia and others. We talk about my teen years, too, when I seemed to love most fiercely, with adolescent hormones surging through me. This was the time of my first passionate love, irresponsible and heady and obsessive.

But instead of nostalgia I begin to re-evaluate.

Is that really what I want or need as a forty-something woman? Adolescent love is also here one minute, gone the next, leaving a heartbroken teen sobbing on the stairs, or, in my daughter's case, watching eighteen series of *Keeping Up with the Kardashians* back-to-back in a dark room until the monoamine chemicals responsible for 'love euphoria' leave her brain.

Falling in love is no longer what I want, perhaps, but walking towards love with my eyes wide open sounds pretty good. A quilt on fire now is not about a polyester duvet, a dozen tea-light candles and a random hook-up. It's conscious intimacy. A growing connection to another human soul.

'Maybe I think of you as a gatekeeper. Like Patti Stanger in *The Millionaire Matchmaker*.'

Luisa looks confused. But doesn't comment.

'The HRT is allowing me to function, and it feels like a window. I feel less anxious now, a bit more like myself. A bit happier. Seeing you helps, and the HRT. But it still feels like something's missing in me. A vital part. And whatever it is, it's making me feel rock bottom. There's something so desperately broken about me and my friends at the moment.'

'There's a lot of research about a midlife slump in happiness, a U-curve. The good news is that it's temporary.' She pauses. 'In most people.'

Dartmouth professor David Blanchflower studied hundreds of thousands of people in 132 countries. He discovered that by sixty you are as happy as you were at eighteen. It is not merely a human phenomenon: great apes experience the curve too, suggesting it's more than simply cultural factors. Chronic depression and despair peak at midlife. There are numerous theories about why this happens: the realisation of mortality, responsibilities, unfulfilled dreams. And the internet is awash with suggestions about tempering this valley: writing lists of gratitude, exercise and healthy food, limiting social media. 'There are plenty of people in their late forties,' says neuroscientist Dean Burnett in *BBC Science Focus* when discussing the U-curve, 'who are having the time of their life.'

I am not having the time of my life. And although I can't voice why, Luisa often does.

Luisa sits back, uncrosses her legs. 'Finding love for yourself is the hardest thing of all. And the most important.'

Perhaps finding love for myself is the key to recovery from this existential angst, but how do I find love for myself when I don't know who I am? I feel like I'm a stranger. To find out who I am would take an energy I haven't got. The drudgery of midlife is a heavy weight. I've never been a morning person. But these days, I find it harder and harder to get out of bed. I ache the moment I first wake, which makes me think my body must ache all through the night. The HRT is helping me with many symptoms, but still, my joints creak and crunch and throb. I make odd clicking noises every time I move, and my teeth hurt. The dentist tells me

I'm grinding my teeth in my sleep, and shows me the edges of my tongue, wavy and grooved. 'You need a mouthguard,' she says. 'And to address anxiety. Have you tried yoga?'

Fuck yoga, I want to shout. But I *have* tried yoga. And running. And weight training. And swimming. But I have no energy for any of it, put in half-hearted attempts, and spend my time watching other, springier women getting it right. Is everyone getting it right? I scroll on Instagram and look at women my age who are shiny and fit and seemingly full of energy. I am judging my insides against other people's outsides, I'm aware, but I can't stop. I tell my teenage daughter to beware of social media, and we discuss the epidemic of mental health issues among her peers, but we don't discuss the epidemic of mental health issues for women in their forties, or the dangers of social media use for those my age. I understand that this culture of perfection is simply an unattainable lie. But still, I look at other women getting it right.

I need to meditate. I need to do yoga. I'm afraid of getting a FitBit as it will shame me. Mostly my exercise consists of constant cleaning up after teens: picking up crap dropped by my children, and I expend a lot of energy in raging at empty cartons put back in the cupboard, empty toilet rolls placed back on the holder, the number of cereal bowls in my daughter's room, and the sweet wrappers I find underneath my son's bed. I don't have energy to exercise, or for 'self-care'.

The administration of parenthood is quite astonishing, and it's exhausting. I have two separate schools sending emails so regularly, and of such utter mundanity, that I miss the important emails among them. Joining the school's parents' WhatsApp group is instantly regrettable. I scan the dozens of messages with an internal rage. Who are these people? Who cares about this stuff? Does nobody work?

And then I feel less than. Maybe I don't care enough? To find out who I am seems unachievable, but I know who I am not. I am not the mother I wanted to be, the mum my children probably want me to be too. I often forget things that most mums surely do not: having milk in the fridge, parents' evening, signing school letters, packed lunchbox snacks. We regularly run out of toilet roll. Twice I have filled the car up with diesel instead of petrol, and three times run out of petrol while driving and the car suddenly chokes, then stops. I have always been a distracted mum, different from the beginning, I realise. A rubbish mother. I remember my daughter, aged four, not wanting to go to school on the second-ever day, her arms around my leg, dragging her into a playground, and in my other arm pulling a sledge with my son, aged two, in his Babygro eating a packet of Monster Munch for breakfast. I remember the looks from the other parents – mums mostly. And one mum, who laughed, and said, 'She's a writer.' But now, perhaps I'm even worse? I'm a writer, a single parent and perimenopausal. They deserve better.

When a well-known tabloid newspaper asks if I'll be photographed and interviewed, along with two other mothers, to head up a campaign to find their 'Mother of the Year', I'm flattered and amused in equal measures. I don't mention it to the children, but when the article is printed, I buy a paper and bring it home to show them at tea-time. The headline is below my photograph: Could You Be Mother of the Year? They put down their forks, slowly, and look at each other. They've always displayed code in this way, a secret language without words that is shared between close siblings. My son's eyebrow raises first. Then my daughter bursts out laughing. Then my son, who laughs so hard he hits the table and holds it to steady himself.

I close the paper and stand up, 'ha ha very funny,' but they don't hear me as they're laughing so hard. I brought this on myself. And it gets worse.

During the weeks following, Mother of the Year becomes my hashtag and the source of all conversations, while my children recount my numerous parental failures and then add the 'Hashtag Mother of the Year' song at the end.

Do you remember the time when you left me in a shoe shop? You had bought some boots – you remembered them – but left me in the shop because you forgot about me. I was SIX weeks old. Hashtag Mother of the Year.

I was the only child in my entire primary school making their own packed lunches. Hashtag Mother of the Year.

You burn everything. Everything we eat tastes of burn. Hashtag Mother of the Year.

I find trying to be Mother of the Year impossible. I'm nowhere near. I love being a mum, and parenting my children is the greatest privilege of my life. But it's never easy.

'I'm thinking of changing my name on the register at school.' My daughter tells me this in a matter-of-fact voice. Then she gets an overwhelmingly powerful look on her face and smiles. 'At sixteen, I am legally allowed to change my name permanently, by deed poll.'

We are eating Japanese food for lunch. I wonder, briefly, if she might be thinking of changing her name to something Japanese – she likes Japanese food – or giving herself a symbol, like Prince, that nobody can ever say.

'Rowan,' she says. 'In case you're wondering.'

I think of my friend named Rowan who my daughter doesn't know and who is kind and funny, beautiful inside and out. 'I know someone awful named Rowan,' I say, out of spite, trying to claw back some sort of power over who she is becoming. And when she doesn't react, I try, 'Isn't one of Boris Johnson's children named Rowan?' Still, no reaction. She smiles, then continues to eat the pickles.

'Why would you change your name?' I blurt out. I can't help myself. I know the parenting rules. I keep my face neutral. Like horses, she seems to smell my fear and happiness. She knows how I'm feeling before I do. I want her to think I'm nonchalant, in the hope that she re-adopts the name I gave her (after both great-grandmothers! I stress), or at least, refrains from changing it permanently. She is reimagining my understanding of that word: permanence. Of course, hardly anything is permanent. Except how much I love her. And how no matter how she changes, she will always be a tiny baby, my Bella, beautiful.

She scowls. 'It's so gendered. Anyway, I own my identity. I have every right to find out who I am. And not be the person you want me to be, but the person I want to be. That I am.'

It terrifies me how perceptive she is, and immature at the same time. I feel stuck in that space and time with her, almost mirroring her adolescence with my own. Yet as she boldly and bravely tries on her identity I feel less courageous. Maybe midlife gives you another chance to try something new that suits you better, that suits you now.

'You could change your name too,' she says.

'I'm very happy with my name,' I tell her. 'And you should be too. Bella is a lovely name.'

She shrugs. 'I'm just more of a Rowan. Not a Bella.' And she's right, a little. My daughter is not the person I imagined in my head. And I'm not the person she imagined either. But neither of us knows the other, I realise, because we don't yet know ourselves. Understandable as a teenager. But not at my age.

We are both changing, inwardly and outwardly. My external appearance is changing even more rapidly than my teen daughter's. My body. In *The Second Sex*, Simone de Beauvoir described bodies as a place in time: 'The body is not a thing, it is a situation: it is our grasp on the world and our sketch of our project.' The two times in our lives that our bodies change so rapidly, adolescence and midlife, are reflecting a changing situation. Or the possibility of one. Perhaps, then, at midlife, as the project of one's life changes rapidly, the sketch of us becomes radically different. It certainly feels as though my body is shouting about identity as much as it was during my teens, expressing the need for an evaluation of my authentic sense of self once more. But I have no answers, only more questions. And the biggest question seems to be this:

Who am I now?

My body feels less of a sketch of my grasp on the world, and more of a crayon scribble by a toddler. Midlife feels less like a crystallising of my sense of self, and more of a losing my identity entirely. I am not remotely polished, grown-up, mature. Despite my best efforts, I am a chaotic disaster, and I have no idea who I am any more. The rapid changes happening to my body, my mind, my soul, make me wonder if I know myself at all, or if I ever have.

I spend a long time looking in the mirror. It's confusing, seeing my face, which seems different every day. Older. I feel like Benjamin Button in reverse. My face is changing so fast I worry that my iPhone face recognition won't identify me. I try and understand what I'm searching for by staring intently at my reflection. A woman's worth in our society is so twisted up and tangled in her appearance. I think of the masks and art and sculptures depicting pregnant, voluptuous and fertile women, the symbols of joy and hope and perhaps purpose. But while I feel increasingly less confident in my appearance, and in my self, as I age, even a bit invisible, do I feel less beautiful? I'm not sure I do. I certainly don't have any desire to look younger than I am. No Botox or fillers for me. I have friends who have faces that quite literally do not move. It scares me so much, the idea of a static face. Faces tell a story, and I worry that smoothing out lines will result in a lost chapter. I also think there is something that I find particularly attractive about older women's faces. I had a hard face as a teen. I had to. I had seen too much already, and looked too streetwise, too cynical. My face now feels softer, laughter lines match the frown lines, and my eyes smile even when my mouth doesn't. My relationship with beauty is changing, along with everything else.

I remember a time working at the cranial facial unit at Great Ormond Street Hospital, where children were disfigured with congenital conditions. Millicent was five when I cared for her and had almost no vision due to an enormous red angry growth covering her face. I spent hours with Millicent, reading *Snow White* at her request. After we read, we would act out the story. She'd have me be the wicked queen and she would be Snow White. She had little vision, but would hold up a mirror and stare at her reflection. 'Mirror, mirror, on the wall, who is the most beautiful of all?' she'd ask.

I wonder if it was helpful, or damaging, for Millicent to chase these ideas of perceived perfection. I wonder about that for all of us.

Increasingly, I find beauty in new places: laughter lines, stretch marks, wrinkles. I look at my hands a lot. My hands after twenty years plus of nursing are as dry and aged as you could imagine, with age spots and wrinkled skin like elephant's hide. 'They look like the hands of a much older woman,' Joy remarks, and sends me special gloves to soak in moisturiser and wear all night, every night. I do not. I love my hands. Every time I see the ageing on them, I see their history. The things I have touched, the other hands I have held. These hands have pressed down on chests, trying to restart hearts. They have caught a baby slipping out of her mum. They have gently washed people who have died, and they have held the hands of their relatives who have lost them. These hands contain all my memories and some that can't be told with words. The lines and wrinkles and marks on them are the language of my hands.

These are the hands that held three children's hands: my step-daughter, my birth daughter, the son I adopted. With these hands I have held the horrors of life, the blood and shit and gunk that makes us human. And the softness of humanity too: my children who held on so tightly to these hands. 'You're all right,' I tell Joy. 'I'll keep these wrinkly old hands for now.'

I am a work in progress. Still learning about what it is that makes us human, what it is that makes us each remarkable. I am looking outward. Nature seems to speak to me more now in my forties than it ever did before. I find myself looking less in the mirror, and more at trees, the sky, the sea. I feel much more abstract, more fluid. This time of feeling unseen, of invisibility, is perhaps not such a negative thing after all. I always imagined that objectification would become less apparent with the loss of youth, perhaps bring an escape from sexualisation. Yet of course, objectification is not limited to the young. Oppression of elderly people from being valued as a contributing responsible adult to becoming dependent – a burden – an object. A sex thing or a sexless thing, both ends of womanhood objectified in different ways. Yet now, I feel neither objectified nor judged, nor observed from the outside. Maybe it is a time to stop people-pleasing, and please myself?

I remember Millicent's laugh and how beautiful she was. In ancient Greek the word for beautiful comes from the word 'hour', and beauty was about 'being of one's hour'. In Latin, beauty 'bellitatem' was a 'state of being pleasing to the senses'. Beauty means being completely and utterly comfortable in my skin.

We are near Barcombe Mills in East Sussex, standing on a river bank. There are five of us, all women, ages ranging from mid-forties to mid-fifties. We are completely naked, comparing bodies. One of the group has had a double mastectomy, another three caesarian sections, while my own abdominal scars are from the removal of a huge ovarian cyst. Scars snake over our collective skin: a faint tracheostomy scar, a road traffic accident, a year of domestic abuse. There are stretch marks like silver fish, and self-harm cuts laddering inner arms and thighs. Our breasts, those of us who have them, are flattened, and we notice that the skin on our knees has dropped for all of us. Our vulvas are wildly different in shape and size and our bodies themselves range from skinny to fat, short to tall. Every one of us complains about our necks, which are crinkly and odd. As Nora Ephron reminded us in *I Feel Bad About My Neck*: 'Anything you think is wrong with your body at the age of thirty-five you will be nostalgic for by the age of forty-five.' We are nostalgic. But although we do not have the same physical worries, we also remember how agonising and painfully self-conscious we were in our younger selves, especially our teens. So we don't complain for long. We get into the river tentatively at first and then in a rush, squealing in delight, lying back and starfishing, letting our heads drop in, hair fanning around us like halos. Teniola shouts: *We are Beautiful*. And so we are.

7

Make the Fucking
Most of It: Death

My Grape Nan (as young children we can't say great) is a small Welsh woman who chain-smokes, lighting a new cigarette as soon as her current one is nearing the end, thereby ensuring she always has one on the go. She has a permanently dour expression and likes to tut instead of using words; her array of disapproving tuts are a language of disappointment. She has what we called (and I inherited): Big Hair Energy, a thick mop of black and grey hair that grows upwards, and she likes to sit cross-legged at my nan's kitchen table, smoking and tutting, and narrowing her eyes if we children are too rowdy. She is almost entirely deaf but refuses to wear hearing aids, and she is divorced – which to my brother and I, aged nine and ten, feels exciting for a woman of her generation, almost exotic – though we can't imagine her ever having been in love. She sleeps in a reclining armchair with the legs raised high, in a living room that has dolls piled floor to ceiling, a lifetime's collection of ceramic creepy dolls with real human hair that are still in boxes, staring out at us. 'Don't play with them,' she says. Tutting. 'They're not toys.' Tom and I love nosing through her bathroom cabinet, at the 'old people stuff': Anusol, Lavender Soap, Denture Cream, three packs of earbuds. There are few clues about her life, before she became an older woman. It is impossible to imagine her laughing, younger, vibrant. And when we come across a photograph of a young, extremely beautiful, smiling-eyed woman, it takes our breath away. 'Is that her?' Tom whispers, wide-eyed. We look at Grape Nan, who has fallen asleep in the chair, her ill-fitting dentures half in half out of her mouth, her snoring louder than I have ever heard (or heard since). It is hard to believe.

Tom and I delight in playing: 'Who Can Wake Her Up?' When Grape Nan sleeps, she is unwakeable. A world war would not rouse her; she famously slept through air raids. Tom and I take turns trying to wake her, clapping over her head, once, banging a stolen-from-school-orchestra cymbal directly over her head. But she is dead to the world, head back, guttural snores. Occasionally my parents leave us with Grape Nan; when we are sick she comes to our house and our parents go off to work, after leaving instructions: soup in the fridge, Calpol and Vicks and calamine lotion on the table, call any problems at all. And we watch as our Grape Nan nods, knowing that the moment Mum leaves she will tut a thousand tuts, wrap our hot bodies in thick dressing gowns and blankets, then position us in front of a three-bar electric fire, so we can 'sweat it out'. She doesn't believe in doctors. 'Quacks,' she says, whenever the word doctor is mentioned or whenever a doctor comes onto the small black and white television. She believes in superstitions and stoicism in equal measures. When I get whooping cough, she suggests taking me to a farm, as 'Everyone knows the only thing that cures it is the breath of a horse.' She is afraid of doctors, but I do remember her saying that she is unafraid of death, just of living. I wonder if it is her profound understanding of the nature of human suffering that makes her a bit difficult; and if living a long lifetime as a woman in our society makes such an understanding of pain and suffering in old age inevitable. My Grape Nan has agency in the face of adversity. Eventually, very old and very tired, she simply says she's had enough of life, as all her friends are dead anyway, and then dies herself a week later.

One of the things that has always fascinated me is that when wards in the hospital are divided between men and women, split into separate areas, with different sets of staff, it is the men's ward where the – predominantly female – nurses want to work. Particularly if the patients are elderly. When I work as a resuscitation nurse I'm forever questioning the other nurses about this. On their ward, the staff rotate every three weeks, from men's to women's wards, then back again. The idea is that this gives them different clinical experience and learning opportunities. However, the manager whispers to me one day that the women's ward is always short-staffed: 'nobody wants to look after the older women. They're a nightmare compared to the men.' It makes me think of my Grape Nan, how complicated she was, her language of tuts, mistrust of 'quacks' and her extreme stoicism – even during a war. Perhaps older women are simply more complex.

'I've run out of blankets and the linen hasn't arrived. On the men's side, I have no issues.' The ward manager continues. 'Mrs Caladine on the women's ward, however, is refusing to get into bed with just a sheet. She spent all night last night sleeping in the chair and said she won't go to bed until her patchwork quilt arrives from the nursing home.'

That evening, I think about Mrs Caladine, how she won't sleep without her handmade blanket, and I read about patchwork quilts. I discover that for centuries, all around the world, women have made art in this way, often communally, coming together from different racial and class backgrounds to tell their stories in fabric. Ralli quilts are traditionally made in Pakistan and western India. They are made by every sector of society including Hindu and Muslim women, and women from different towns or villages or tribes, with the colours and designs varying among these groups. The name comes from 'ralanna', a word meaning to mix or connect. I find the names of the stitching patterns and the fine decorative stitches of quilts poetic: *broken plaid; hanging diamond; twisted rope; true lover's knot*. The names of the patterns of quilt making, in Amish culture, for example, sometimes ring with power: *streak of lightning*. And the language of quilting is sometimes literal: during pioneer days, in the early American west, women would save letters from home, postcards and newspaper clippings and sew them into their patterns, stitching their lives into history.

I read about remarkable quilters. Harriet Powers was born into slavery in rural Georgia. She recorded local legends, Bible stories and astronomical events on her quilts, connecting art and science in a way that still feels urgent. Nancy Crow, a contemporary American quilter, describes the expansive nature of the art form: 'The purpose of my quilts is to make something beautiful but, at the same time, my quilts are a means of expression, representing my deepest feelings and my life experiences. In addition, my quilts are all about how I see colour and colour relationships, how I see shapes, and how I see line and linear movements. They are also about complexity, sadness, and hope.'

Now in my forties, I increasingly feel rich with complexity, sadness and hope. I've been thinking a lot about the older women in my family, the generations before me, and how we view ageing in our culture. In some countries, menopause is seen as gaining literal supernatural powers that lead to the increased bargaining ability of elderly women in their communities and households. Older women are not only seen and heard, they are revered and respected. Post-menopausal women in some parts of West Africa, those from Fon, Ewe, Adja and Yoruba cultures for example, are seen as spiritually gifted, and able to whisper to gods and ancestors, connecting with the past and with other worlds. Contrastingly, in the UK the 'anti-ageing' brand is big business. Ageing is a dirty word. What might we learn from other cultures? There is so much negativity and stigma in our own, attached to speaking openly and positively about changes at this time of life. And yet we are doing so many things later and later – establishing careers, marriages, parenting – that it can come as a total surprise when meno-pause crashes in. In too many cultures, women are almost forbidden to age, and are encouraged to be fearful of ageing. Indeed, the anti-ageing market in the US is valued at over 44 million dollars. Are the perimenopausal and menopausal symptoms we experience themselves a form of internalised ageism? Because the relationship between their prevalence and severity and the correlation of them with the prejudice and discrimination against older people in those same coun-tries surely cannot be a coincidence.

I do wonder if this has this always been the case or if it is that we, as a society, no longer respect our elders as we once did. I would like to know how those older generations of women got over the hump of midlife messiness, and if the hump was as big and if not, why not? If they experienced peri-menopause, this unspoken thing, what form did it take? I want to know what the experience of my Grape Nan was – and if she had a language for it at all. I wonder what they would make of wellness, and 'reclaiming our bodies', and black cohosh tea and the movement of openness towards sex and dating and the menopause. I wonder what they would make of the HRT patches that one in ten women in the UK now rely on, like me. My Grape Nan is gone, but when I talk to her daughter – my nan – about her menopause, she sits back and tells me the story of going to her army doctor, thinking she was pregnant – at thirty-nine years old. The doctor told her: 'you're not pregnant, you're going through the change.' I ask if she had symptoms, how it felt.

'Nothing,' she says. 'I never had a period ever again. Thought I was pregnant!'

But then later she describes sitting next to my granddad and being so hot that she felt as if she were burning in a fire. And Granddad watching her change colour from white to pink to red. 'He called me a raspberry ripple ice-cream,' she laughs.

I'm interested in the older generation's experience of midlife in relation to what is increasingly being termed in mainstream media as 'the menopause revolution'. Diane Danzebrink runs the menopause support network and describes far too many women as 'needlessly suffering in silence'. I think about the female nurses I work with, so many of them at midlife, going through menopause while working long night shifts, or twelve-and-a-half-hour days, often dressed in PPE, with limited breaks, or too often, none at all. We don't hear from these women. What we do hear, again and again, are stories about women who have had terrible experiences trying to get their voices heard and the treatment they need and deserve. Carolyn Harris, a Labour MP introducing legislation seeking to overhaul menopause rights, justifiably said in the House of Commons that 'generation after generation of women have been let down, or simply thrown on the scrap heap as a result of the menopause.'

My nan, however, doesn't consider her midlife a time of suffering. She sees it instead as a time of change, as much a positive as a negative; a period of profound reckoning, a part of the fabric of life. Another patch in the quilt. When I ask my nan about Grape Nan and all the other women of that generation, whether they had symptoms, how they managed, she can't recall anyone going through anything, other than simply 'changing'. 'We are young and then we are old. Happens almost overnight really.' While she is talking about The Change, I wonder if that's actually a better term than menopause. The shock is that it is a shock in the first place. I am far from the first woman to go through it, or talk, or shout about it, and yet

it feels like it. This universal experience that binds together
women everywhere throughout history and time seems to be
zeitgeisty, and yet it is older and perhaps more profound than
I can comprehend. It feels deeper than medical, a kind of spiritual change. At first, I thought it was a time of becoming
afraid, but increasingly I feel the opposite: it is a time of
becoming *less* afraid. And this process of change hurts in my
body, and my mind and soul. This shedding of fear, as well as
youth and fertility, like a snake shedding skin, is, for me, a
painful evolving into enlightenment. A time to sit in the mystery of women's bodies, of time, of life and humanity itself. A
reflection and pause before embodiment of urgency as well as
acceptance and agency. A surrender of sorts to the idea that I
know nothing, less than before. This moving away from concrete ideas to abstract thinking indeed feels climacteric, and as
though I'm climbing a ladder towards freedom. I feel simultaneously incredibly fragile and amazingly strong.

In *How to Stay Sane in an Age of Division*, Elif Shafak describes real change as happening in the spaces between: 'We
must strive to become intellectual nomads, keep moving, keep
learning, resist confining ourselves in any cultural or mental
ghetto, and spend more time not in select centres but at the
margins, which is where real change comes from.' Women are
always fluid, and often live in the in-between spaces, as do

writers. The margins are not empty, but the space is a place of change and possibility and adaptability. Perhaps midlife is the biggest space of all, the widest margin. In any case, the mid-point, the space in the margins, feels like a time when we have room to imagine our endings. A time of surrender to the uncertain nature of life and the universe, one where I realise that the control I had over my life never really existed in the first place. I think often of the middle point of writing a book, particularly a novel. Editors warn of the 'soggy middle', a time in a narrative where the story has a solid beginning and end but less attention has been paid to the important middle section. And of course, it is in the middle section where the bulk of the story, the main character development, the meaning of the work is found. The centre of a story is the hottest part of a flame. The point around which everything else revolves. Where everything before is certain and nothing afterwards is known. The most human time of all.

Ellen Langer, a Harvard professor, studies control. In 1975, in an article published by the *Journal of Personality and Social Psychology*, she coined the term 'illusion of control'. She used it to describe how we often perceive we have autonomy and can control external (and sometimes internal) events and yet the reality is that often, we cannot. We can't reverse ageing, whatever 'anti-ageing' marketing campaigns tells us. We can't stop dying. We are blown around by the wind of fate and time, and very little we can do ourselves will alter that. Perhaps this time – like the perimenopause – is for reflection, re-evaluation, and a search for new identity. A time when we are forced to accept that we can't control most things, and we do not know what is coming our way, there is only right now. You and I and everyone reading this will one day simply be a story, like the story of my Grape Nan. We can't control the story in the way we'd like. But we can make it more textured. Life is a mixture of tragedy and joy for all of us, but it is perhaps in tragedy that we grow and learn the most. If play is the work of children, coming to terms with loss is the work of adults. Losing my mind, body and sense of self is traumatic but increasingly, far worse, I am losing people I love. Yet with each loss comes a beautiful, terrible wisdom, a richness to my own story. I am beginning to appreciate that growing old is hard, but it's also a privilege that too many people don't get to experience.

I am with my teenage daughter, walking towards the exit after a literary talk. She hangs back, and I feel her hot breath on my neck. I turn to see her face: she is afraid. A woman is walking towards us. Staggering, limping, dragging her foot and leaning on another woman. She introduces herself as Caroline. I can see why my usually fearless daughter is afraid. She is not used to seeing dying up close. And yet I am. Nurses are. Death is a sensory experience. To watch a person dying is usually pretty unremarkable, even during the final moments. Things get softer, slower, calmer. But the other senses are assaulted, no matter how natural the situation, how dignified. Like many nurses, I have touched and smelled and tasted death. I've heard the many soundtracks of dying, the unexpected death track of alarms, of screaming, crying wrongness. The distant beat of a slowing heart. The shape of air squeezed through a broken body, an off-key pitch. I hear it immediately. Caroline has yellow-tinged skin and when she breathes she rasps, every breath crunching. Her eyes are hollow and sunken, and she has a hugely distended swollen abdomen. She moves slowly but there's an urgency about the way she speaks, as though every word matters. 'I am dying,' she tells my daughter. 'Don't look so worried,' she says. 'It's a part of life.' She is so matter of fact about dying that I can feel my daughter relax. Emotions jump through her skin and into mine. Caroline is almost upbeat. She tells me her thoughts about the talk I have just given, and the nurses she has met, good and bad, and she laughs a bit too. But the horror of her failing body, the pain I see flash across her face intermittently, is hard to imagine. She is fifty-eight years old.

There are many ways to live, and there are many ways to die. As a nurse I've seen them all. There appears, too often, to be no parallel between the way a person lives, the character, what they bring to the table, and how they die. The greatest tragedies seem to fall at the doors of the best people. The nicest families face the worst struggles. And the meanest people can live forever. Death doesn't care about your character, whether you've been good or kind or evil. It is indiscriminate. Unconditional love exists as does unconditional death. Like love, it can feel as if we have no control of that part of us and some people are simply lucky enough to manage dignity and peace at the end of their lives. Both death and love can mean peace or they can mean tragedy. And neither outcome is always a reflection of the life a person lived. Caroline lives a good life.

I visit Caroline at her flat in Nottingham; her home is filled with flowers and there are posters on the walls, mostly of art exhibitions, colourful, vibrant, bohemian. We sit in the small terrace garden for as long as she can stand the light and heat and then move into her bedroom, where she lies down, and I perch on the end of her bed, closing the curtains a fraction. Her dressing table is covered in pots of tablets, a neon yellow sharps bin, syringes of all sizes, gloves, dressing packs. My eyes scan the tablets: my nurse brain can tell by the types of medication and the doses how long Caroline might have left, or at least, how long her medical team think she has. Not long.

'I'll be sleepy soon,' she says, 'the pain meds are kicking in. So ask me anything you want.' She's invited me here to her

home in order to share her story and give much-needed balance to mine. I jump at the chance to hear her perspective,
what it actually feels like at the end. Yet even with my years of
clinical experience, I am a little afraid, because I am not here
as a nurse, but as a witness. I think of all the things we say in
our lives, our conversations about nothing, how little we talk
about the deep things. I wonder if we use language as a protective avoidance, our chatter a distraction from all things
painful, real. She turns around on her side, unable to get comfortable. I try and help her but she swats me away. Her
abdomen is grotesquely distended; she looks nine months
pregnant.

I think about what I can learn from her. A nurse asking a
patient for advice about what illness means may appear odd,
but to do so – to ask people about their 'lived experience' of
illness and disease – is part of a growing movement accepting
that as health professionals, we are looking from the outside
in. And the only way to truly understand pain and suffering is
from the inside.

But we don't talk long about her dying experience. It seems
to me that as people are dying, when they know they have
reached the end of their lives, every word matters. Language
itself changes in the dying, the meaning of words, how we form
them, why. Perhaps living with death makes the story more
important. Because our stories are what we leave behind.

Instead of dying we talk about Caroline's stories. The room is full of them. I read aloud 'The Veteran', a Dorothy Parker poem she has framed over her bed:

> When I was young and bold and strong,
> The right was right, the wrong was wrong.
> With plume on high and flag unfurled,
> I rode away to right the world.
> But now I'm old – and good and bad,
> Are woven in a crazy plaid.
> I sit and say the world is so,
> And wise is he who lets it go.

Caroline talks of her passion for Dorothy Parker. And poetry. And I hear about her past loves and her family and her travels and adventures. She says nothing of her work or the things she has owned. Who really cares about all that, in the end. I do ask her, though, about regrets. 'I wish I'd worried less,' she says. 'About stupid stuff. And danced more. Shouted a bit. If I had my time over, I'd read more books, take more walks in the rain. Have tons more sex. Watch plays, and theatre. How I'd love to go to the theatre now.' She is getting tired, I can see. I jot down what she says and close my notebook. She asked that I write about her and since then, I have been waiting to find the perfect moment to do so. And it is when I find myself asking the question, How on Earth Will I Get to Sixty, that I think of Caroline. And of what a privilege it is to get older. Perhaps it is only at midlife that we can glimpse death in order to grasp on to life. Caroline's real love is of life itself. 'We are not here long for this earth,' she tells me as I leave. 'Make the fucking most of it.'

The reasons for living have been at the heart of the arts throughout history. Whether art is for beauty or politics or simply escapism, the best of it explores the question of what it means to be human, in that place, in that time. The universe feels at once timeless but also random, an organised chaos. Art can be a mirror that shows us the true reflection of ourselves. I have no doubt that it is medication keeping Caroline alive, but it is art that gives her remaining days meaning. To understand film, dance, theatre, visual art, creative writing is to understand suffering. And an understanding of suffering can alleviate it.

Science has very little explanation for menopause, so I begin to search in art for what it means to be midlife. I want to understand if there is a way of thinking philosophically about the physical effects that accompany the hormonal changes and loss of fertility in our perimenopause. Why does our bone density change? What is it preparing us for, this lightness of being? The message of midlife in science seems to be one of unexplained theories of evolutionary biology or a simplistic medicalised model of (white, able-bodied) anatomy, but perhaps art has another answer? I read the classics, stand in front of the most beautiful paintings, attend theatre performances and try and absorb as much culture as possible. But it's not in high-brow culture that I find the most meaning about death and life, and this, the mid-point in between.

In the late eighteenth century, a period that historian Richard Holmes refers to as 'the Age of Wonder', scientists and artists were knocking around together sharing ideas. If ours is a time of polarisation and division and echo chambers, theirs was quite the opposite. Astronomer William Herschel – who discovered, among other things, the planet Uranus – was great friends with the famously hell-raising Romantic poet Lord Byron. After a lifetime of groundbreaking scientific discoveries, a memorial stone at Westminster Cathedral commemorates Herschel, on which are the Latin words: 'He broke through the barriers of the heavens.' It is perhaps the pivot point of the balance between sceptical analysis and profound mystery that allowed Hershel and so many artists and scientists of that era to break through barriers, to find meaning in giant questions. But they also had enormous fun. William Herschel had a forty-foot telescope built in Slough, inside which Byron famously threw him a champagne party.

Surrounding myself with a diverse set of friends who think differently to me feels like a worthy way to delve deeper into my own situation and the bigger questions of life. And we have a lot of fun, too. My friends and I are at a street food festival, the kind where you pay £6 for a single taco and drink warm beer until you are forced to use the disgusting toilets. Everyone in this place is around twenty years younger than us. They seem to be cooler than us, having quiet, sober conversations around upside-down barrels being used as tables. My middle-aged women friends and I are not quiet. Emma, as ever, is dancing provocatively, and is flashing her 'new bra, do you like it?' at the man selling ramen. We spot another friend, who joins in, bringing more women our age over until we have taken over the bar area, pushing out the chic young people to the periphery. They watch us as though we are a circus show. I overhear one of the younger men who leans towards a young woman, nods our way and says: tragic.

Our antics may seem tragic to that couple. But we are not tragic. Tragic is the fact that Orla will be going in on Tuesday for a hysterectomy, that Teniola is nursing her 101-year-old granddad at home and hasn't been out of the house for months, Sarah's husband asked for a divorce last week, and she is dealing with a suicidal, self-harming teenager. Tragic is when, halfway through the night, Sarah leans on my shoulder in the disgusting toilet and tells me her fourteen-year-old has now been sectioned following another suicide attempt. 'Do you want me to drop you at home?' I say. And she shakes her head so hard her earrings make a jangling noise. 'No way. I need this. It's fresh air.' And the air in that toilet is anything but fresh but I know exactly what she means. It's not the heavy drinking either – although we all *appear* hammered, at least three of us are driving, and Samira is an alcoholic and tee-total. She's having the most fun of all, flirting with the younger men and handing out her number to a good-looking stranger for no-strings-attached sex. 'It doesn't have your name on it,' he says. 'Does it matter,' she replies. Later they disappear into the disgusting toilet together. And we watch the line get longer and longer, people becoming more impatient until they emerge, red-faced, sweaty and stinking. This is not how I would have imagined a lollipop lady from Tunbridge Wells behaving at the age of fifty. But I'm not sure entirely what it was I did imagine. Someone on a stall selling fairy cakes at the school fete? Those things are equally true. But we are complex and messy and contain many threads. Being with my friends always makes me think of the Age of Wonder, and the import-ance of paradox and sometimes raucous fun in a serious world. We might not be having champagne parties in tele-scopes, but we wear many hats, to the benefit, I think, of each of our identities. We are multiplicity. Responsible, silly, adult, immature, debauched, professional, sewn together in equal measures with the thread of this life, this time, this moment in history.

Later, we queue outside a fried chicken shop in Lewisham and chat to strangers, fellow waifs and strays, and it occurs to me that maybe we are all waifs and strays and that's OK. Better than OK. None of us is fine. Maybe nobody in the world is fine. But there is a myth of both middle age and of motherhood, that women at midlife have their shit together, and are the glue of society, the dependable ones. And that is true in many ways. But we are often not fine, together. There are chinks in the armour of our responsible selves, and I am learning that these chinks are not defects, but rather, coping strategies. To let in the light. And now and again, these moments of hedonistic debauchery hold us up, even as we are falling over. We dance and mess around and talk shit all night until the dawn. And I understand that the shit we are talking is not shit at all; it's the underneath. The fabric of us. The wild hearts of who we are and what's happening in our lives. It's therapy. And it's not about drinking or late nights or fun, it's about togetherness and friendship and absolutely about sharing struggles. I love the frank conversations I have with my friends and with strangers when stripped of sensibilities and responsibilities just for a brief moment.

'Do you think we're having a midlife crisis?' I ask Joy.

Dante Alighieri in the *Divine Comedy* described midlife in a way I relate to: 'In the middle of the journey of our life I came to myself within a dark wood where the straight way was lost. Ah, how hard a thing it is to tell what a wild, and rough, and stubborn wood this was, which in my thought renews the fear!'

We are in a dark wood together.

'Not a crisis, no. None of us is buying motorbikes or hooking up with twenty-two-year olds.'

'Speak for yourself,' Samira is coming out of the chicken shop carrying a few boxes. She passes them around to each of us. 'And I'm not talking about motorbikes.'

'It's a time of realisation.' Joy bites into a chicken leg. She's a real foodie and gets organic vegetables delivered weekly, and keeps beloved chickens for fresh eggs, yet is also the biggest fan of greasy fried chicken. 'It feels like we've all lived a certain way up until now. Focused on stuff, you know, the dream of a wedding, two point four children and Having it All. Great careers, perfect bodies, perfect relationships, spectacular homes. And then this perimenopause hits us in the face and tears all that apart.'

'I feel like I'm falling apart, it's true,' I say.

Joy laughs. 'It means we're awake. Fully shaken awake even if we don't choose it. And now we get to reset if we want. I don't have to live the life I thought I wanted. I was told I wanted by society. I mean I can choose, actually choose to be standing here with you lot in the middle of the night talking crap and eating crap.'

'I'm scared but I'm grateful at the same time,' says Samira. 'I mean, yes, I feel like I'm falling apart, but I also feel like I can put myself back together the way I want. On my own terms. I know who I am or at least, I know who I want to be. And it's not what I thought at all, what I was told by society and culture and the patriarchy. The only voice I care about listening to right now is my own.'

Joy nods. 'I don't need to wait for everything to be perfect to be happy. When everything looked perfect, I was unhappy. Now everything is a mess, I feel happier.'

I've been lucky enough in my career and life to meet some of the best thinkers and change-makers: writers, artists, scientists, academics, medics. But it is in late-night conversations with my wayward friends where I have always found the most wisdom. I find meaning in art, in science, in philosophy. And sometimes, in the 4 a.m. queue for a chicken shop.

'I feel a bit broken,' I say.

'You're not broken.' Joy bites into another piece of chicken. 'You're broken open.'

8

Women are Water, as Well as Fire: Beauty

My daughter and I are standing opposite each other in her bedroom, both of us puffy-faced and crying. I hardly ever go into her bedroom. I rarely, these days, even see the children. They emerge every now and then to eat, heads down, ignoring my attempts at conversation. They text me or WhatsApp me from upstairs: *What's for dinner?* Or, *I'm going out on Friday.* But today, I find a handwritten note: *I'm getting my septum pierced. I'm not asking you for permission. I'm doing it anyway.* Her floor is covered in dirty washing, cereal bowls and glasses. There's a small pet feeding bowl – with puppy paw print pattern all over it – that I don't recognise and don't dare ask about.

My son is hiding, as he always does, when he sees that I'm about to lose my shit.

'If you don't pick up your washing and tidy your room you will not be going on the school trip,' I shout. 'I'm sick of it.'

I think about the possibility of going on complete strike. I wonder how long it would take them to realise. I imagine them trying to squeeze more and more laundry into the basket, and somehow get the lid on, the thought of putting a wash on not crossing their minds in the slightest. That morning I find two empty milk cartons carefully placed back in the fridge, an unflushed toilet, a sink full of washing up and an empty cereal box put back in the cupboard. I find toenail clippings on the bathroom cabinet, and wet towels all over my son's floor.

'You think I have time for this?' I shout. Both my daughter and I mirror each other, waving our arms around expressively, almost violently. We are so similar, it scares us both. 'What do you think I do all day? Sit around?'

She scowls. 'I didn't ask to be born.' Then: 'I am going to get my septum pierced, whether you like it or not.'

I pause and take a breath. 'Just try it. I *dare* you.'

We stare at each other, unblinking, trying to find words that will hit the other harder. Eye contact between parent and child is a language that goes from learning to trust as a baby, to challenging that trust as a teen. Most of our healthy conversations happen on car journeys, or when we are walking side by side. I always assumed that was about my daughter not wanting to look into my eyes, to feel safer somehow in a layer of false anonymity. But I wonder if it's a two-way process. My expectations of them have never been overreaching. I always wanted for them to be as healthy and happy as possible, but always for them to know they are loved no matter what. My expectations of myself as a parent have grown with them, however, and stretched out into long shadows. The psychoanalyst and paediatrician Donald Winnicott stated in *Playing and Reality* that parenting should simply be 'good enough'. I've always subscribed to that, but these days it feels more like 'just about good enough' – and even then, some days it feels entirely lacking.

'It's my body,' she says. 'You do not own my body. I could pierce anything I want, and you can't do anything about it.' She lifts her head high, waiting for my pain and horror, a winning smile crosses her lips. She will soon be an adult, in between spaces too, struggling with her own identity at the same time as I am. We are in a gap together, flailing around. Life is not linear, it's circular. And we're currently at the opposite, same points.

I try not to react. But my own rage matches hers, as ever. You can feel rage in the atmosphere, heavy and smelling of pepper.

'I didn't teach you the time,' I say. 'When you were little. I didn't teach you the time.' My voice gets louder, loud enough that my son comes in after all, and stands watching us, as we compete with each other as to who has done the worst thing. 'I purposefully didn't teach you to tell the time. No clocks. Nothing.' I am shouting again now, 'even though you had to learn it for maths. I didn't want you knowing what time it was so I could sometimes put you to bed earlier than bedtime. So I could lie and say it was seven when it was really only six-thirty. One time it was six.'

I stop shouting. Look at them both, their mouths dropping open.

I wake with insomnia that is hormonal and also an all-consuming existential fear. HRT at least reduces the insomnia. HRT seems to be the only thing that is just about keeping me going. But the HRT patches that I have come so quickly to rely upon are among the things that pharmacists run out of fairly regularly. Women are low on the priority list, as ever. The pharmacist shakes his kindly head slowly; the patches have not arrived yet. There's a shortage. Brexit, he shrugs.

After a few days running dangerously close to completely running out, I visit three separate chemists. One of them produces something like the patches I have been using, but not quite the same.

'Same thing,' he assures me as I suspiciously glance at the box. 'Same ingredients.'

The box is a different shape entirely, and the patches are smaller. 'I really need my normal dose. More, probably.'

He smiles. 'This is all we can get at the moment.'

So I take it. But the patches keep falling off. Usually my patches survive sweat, baths, showers, materials rubbing against them, all manner of things. But these patches peel off then disappear, and I find scrunched-up plastic HRT patches around the house, menopausal breadcrumbs. I am panicked. I won't get a repeat prescription this soon. I am only supposed to change the patch every three or four days, but I'm having to stick a new one on daily. Am I absorbing mega amounts of medication? I am barely hanging on and surely it's these small patches that enable me to get up and function.

It is evening when I am reaching for a top shelf glass when my daughter says What. The. Fuck. She's taken to swearing like a drunken pirate.

I turn. 'Stop swearing. I mean it, it's disrespectful, and some people get really offended by it and if you start swearing as a matter of course, sooner or later you'll be swearing all the time.' I tell her this even though I too can swear like a pirate. Hypocrisy belongs to parenthood.

She rolls her eyes. And her head. 'Sorry.'

'I mean it. And it's a lazy use of language. Anyway, why did you say it?'

She calls her brother. They stand across the kitchen from me. 'Raise your arms,' she says.

I have no idea what she's talking about, but I know well enough that sometimes it's just easier and quicker to obey random requests than get into a long discussion. I raise my arms, thinking my jumper must have something on it, under the armpits. Deodorant stains. A rip.

My son is cracking up. My daughter looks like I'm mad. 'You've lost it. What even is that?'

I look down at the exposed skin on my waist, and laugh. A large thick circle of neon green around my entire middle. 'Oh. My HRT patch kept falling off. So I taped it. Only we didn't have any duct tape, only Frog Tape – the masking tape for painting.'

'You've Frog Taped hormones to your stomach,' she whispers. My son is still laughing, snorting and pointing his finger at me like I'm a court jester. But my daughter's eyes open wider with embarrassment every day. 'It's a new low,' she says, scowling. 'A new low.'

Stella Duffy, a writer and psychotherapy researcher, describes ageing as an embodied existential experience, not the medicalised model that narrates menopause as a problem, HRT as a solution. It does feel as if I'm having an internal existential experience, and yet other than the HRT I'm already so reliant on, I don't know how to solve myself. I am struggling with the space Margaret Drabble describes in *The Middle Ground* as, 'the middle years, caught between children and parents, free of neither: the past stretches back too densely, it is too thickly populated, the future has not yet thinned out.' But did previous generations of women struggle as much as I seem to be?

Neither my mum nor my grandmothers had – as far as I know, or they will reveal to me – any major symptoms. They did not have HRT. But they did speak of their changing. When I turned forty my nan told me on the phone, 'I had my menopause at your age,' but I laughed. I look back at my laughing, at my thinking it was funny that she told me. That it somehow was a joke. That it would never happen to me, and it must have been a generational fluke. I wasn't listening to her at all. Older generations of women didn't say as much, but perhaps they listened harder. Maybe they understood better what was in the things left unsaid, the silences, the gaps. Language and communication between women change with each generation, morph and shift with the social constructs around us, the shape of technology, as well as political mood. But it's also deeper than that. Women's relationships with each other, their shared experience of a collective womanhood, has shifted and become much more individualistic, along with everything else.

The sisterhood has always existed. My friends and I are good at talking. We speak in a candid, frank and sometimes gratuitous way. We are proud of this; at least I am. My daughter's generation are even more this way, perhaps, developing language that is much more inclusive, tolerant and kind (to each other, at least. . .), requiring more words, new vocabulary and phrases and less slang or shortcuts. I often imagined that my mum's and especially my nan's generations of women were expected to 'put up and shut up', but didn't think too much about how women are fluid. It is rivers that cut through rocks. Women have always been water, as well as fire.

Research suggests that the last of the senses to leave us as we die is our hearing. Perhaps it is listening, really listening, that connects us to each other more than anything else. Even our unconscious bodies are searching for the words. Our need for voices, for understanding, for stories.

I didn't listen to my nan. It wasn't a warning when she told me about her menopause coming early. It was a quiet message. In her voice was a gentle calm, a reassurance. She wasn't trying to shock or scare me, or make me laugh. She was talking to me about life, telling me something about the nature of time, and of womanhood. I can hear her words now, if I listen really carefully to the silence and things she left unsaid:

You will be old like me one day, if you're lucky, and you too will be looking back. You are forty now. Halfway to where I am. The mid-point. My change happened right then. The stepping towards wisdom, towards understanding my body and my life, towards finding meaning in this world, this universe, and acceptance that in just a moment, a blink, I'll be an old woman, looking back, telling a granddaughter who is changing: Look here – I changed too.

Take good care of your time. It will all go too fast. Life changes overnight.

*

I am standing in the mortuary of the Nightingale Hospital, looking at the rows of shipping containers in the empty warehouse, which is a bit like an aircraft hangar. The shipping containers that we understand will soon be full of bodies. Having left the nursing register in 2018 I never expected to return to clinical work. Even in those early days when the pandemic first emerged, I joke with the friends who text to ask if I am dusting off my uniform. 'Not unless the world is about to end. Two kids, single parenting, full-time writing work. Peri-bloody-menopause. No chance. We're barely holding on by a thread as it is.' And it often feels like that, although the rush of love I often feel from my children, my family, my friends, is more glue than thread.

But then it seems as if the world is about to end.

I sign up to the emergency Covid-19 Temporary Register and am doing refresher training at Guy's and St Thomas hospital. I plan to split my time between St Thomas' and the newly built Nightingale Hospital. In due course, Boris Johnson is admitted to the intensive care unit at St Thomas' with Covid. I decide to give that ward a wide berth, for many reasons. Instead, I am on the Compassionate Care team. My job title seems to change on a daily basis: today, I am Lead Nurse for Compassionate Care, yesterday, Head of Nursing for Compassionate Care, tomorrow, Lead Nurse for end-of-life care. It feels like an important job, compassion. We are told that our single function in the NHS, at this time, is to save as many lives as possible. Yet we are not saving lives, not nearly as many as we want. Perhaps that makes compassion matter even more. How compassionate we are to each other, in this, is how history will judge us. And it's how history should judge us. All of my jobs involve many different teams of many different people: end-of-life care, bereavement, family support and liaison office, the chaplaincy and the mortuary. I'm on the periphery of all of them, with far more experienced and expert people running the show; I often feel more of a hindrance than a help. I don't feel qualified to be lead or head of any sort of nursing, at least not this, but I'm trying to learn what this is, what I'm here for, and what my part is, in this slice of living history. We are all trying to make sense of things. Externally the world is changing, it's on fire, and it's hard to disentangle internal and external thoughts, and we are so connected to everything, and everyone.

Ageing, and how we think of older people, has become a central concern, due to the lack of concern expressed by those in charge. Despite the narrative politicians repeat about a 'protective ring' around our care homes, our nursing homes, housing predominantly older people, it is those elderly who are dying in vast numbers. It is elderly people in our society who are disregarded, inadequately protected, left to die horrendous, lonely and desperate deaths from this awful disease.

I visit my nan, who is shielding and in her late nineties, disabled and completely alone in her house. I take a bag of her favourite foods: Walkers prawn cocktail crisps, melon slices, a scotch egg, a small trifle. She is leaning out of the window, which is wide open, and I stand across the path, mask on; we can't hear each other well. Instead, we just look at each other and wave frantically, as though she's on a ship leaving for a long journey to a far-flung destination. Or maybe I am. I wave until my arm starts hurting. 'I love you,' I shout. And she shouts 'I love you' back. Then, I catch, 'Don't worry about me, love. I'll be all right.' I am panicked all the way home, thinking of her alone. Still, we are lucky. In these first weeks of the pandemic elderly people are sent back to care homes without being tested for Covid, superspreaders to their friends and neighbours, a damning insight into just how little older people are valued in this Darwinian system. Of course, the public painful outcry does not mirror the political silence. These older people dying in care homes are each somebody's mother, uncle, grandfather. Somebody's nan. The pandemic has uncovered for many people the pandemics that existed already. And it also uncovers the pandemic of ageism.

These are chilling times. My body, meanwhile, is burning up. It is red hot. I am burning. I have to visit the mortuary now and again, and when I do, I spend more time here than is probably necessary. I wonder if I am trying to shake myself into the enormity of the situation. We do not know what is coming. We only know for sure that it will be big, and it will be bad. There are many shipping containers. I look at them all and imagine a loved one inside them, alone in this draughty, desolate and artificial place. My friends and family flash in front of me. I can't stop thinking about my children, alone and likely terrified, waiting for me to return and hoping I don't bring back a deadly disease with me. It is very early days in this, and we all believe in the possibility that we might die. It's hard to imagine dying, even while we live in its shadow. I'm desperately searching for an understanding of Covid, and of death and dying. I am in shock, like everyone else. A bit numb with it. But also, I realise, as I stand in the cold air of the only place in the makeshift field hospital that is deliberately kept freezing, I am searching for cool air. Alongside fear and sadness, I find relief in this ice cold. The enormity of my love for my children, and theirs for me, fills even this space. I stand here in this makeshift mortuary. This unreal space, that is most real. The world is alight with anxiety, the rug pulled from beneath our feet. Whatever happens, nothing will be the same again. Yet here, everything is icy silent. A cold, quiet nothingness. A blank page.

It is here in the mortuary that I check my phone. Emma has sent her daily video clip, of her dancing in her pyjamas, loud music blaring out. Stripper dance moves, sometimes with a disco ball in the background. Once, a smoke machine. She doesn't text. Nothing poignant or heartfelt. No words of worry or declarations of friendship and love. Just Emma being Emma, reminding me that my friends are always with me, and she is utterly alive in this place and time of death.

I come home late, driving through the empty streets, crying all the way. Often I phone Joy, and sob. And she just listens to me crying. I think of our mundane conversations in the past, about dating and gossip and the drudgery of parenting teens. And we have no words for this now, but we have language anyway. After I cry a bit, sometimes she cracks a joke. *The universe is having a midlife crisis now. At least we're not alone.* We reminisce about The Before.

'Do you remember the time I burnt my chest by using suncream in one area only to write the name of a man?'

'That time I brought your uniform to London Bridge station, and you got changed for work in a portaloo, having been out all night.'

'I remember your dad trying to surf in India, heading into the biggest wave you ever saw, fearless.'

I picture my dad. Wonder what he would have made of this Time of Times. We are all heading, unwillingly, into this towering wave. And we are afraid. But it helps to hear Joy's voice. To hear her silence too. The things unsaid, that we both hear.

When I get home, it's night and the house is dark. A fox looks at me from the bins, and saunters away. I have no idea when bin day is, or will be. In months gone by this would have stressed me out. Funny the things we worry about.

Before leaving the car, I wipe everything down with flash wipes – even the handle of the car. Then, on the doorstep, I take off my shoes, name badge and keys, and wipe those. I shout through the letter box: *Rooms*. And hear distant thudding of footsteps on the stairs. Inside, I walk straight to the kitchen, and the washing machine, and strip off, throwing in all my clothes on a hot wash. I then wash my hands for a long time, wash them again. I spray down my shoes, keys, phone. I quickly head upstairs where it is quiet. And I imagine them on the other sides of their bedroom doors, waiting. I glance at my face. Red and angry, and puffy from tears. Then shower, washing my hair twice.

And then I pray to all the gods.

Please don't let me give my children this virus.

I dry myself off, put on a dressing gown and emerge. 'You can come out now.'

My mum taught me kindness, and radical empathy, and anxiety in equal measures. She taught me that it is vulnerability that makes us human. We are all so vulnerable, yet Covid is dehumanising in many ways. Most of the patients in Covid intensive care are proned, that is, lying face down. There are no visiting family members to give those details that make us, about relationships, work, passions, history. The staff are head to toe in PPE, also faceless. And over the chugging machinery and alarms, behind masks, no voices either. No faces. No voices. There are rows and rows of beds, opposite each other, each proned patient surrounded by machinery, ventilators, syringe drivers, drip stands, blood transfusions. On the monitors a person's insides make numbers and patterns and tell the nurses what the oxygen levels are, the pattern of electricity in a heart, the arterial blood pressure. If scrolling through Instagram encourages me to judge my insides against another person's outsides, then this is the opposite of that. Looking at the monitor I know I am blessed. So lucky, to be standing, and – hopefully – Covid-free thus far. The act of breathing itself, feels like a privilege.

I am talking to the doctor in charge of the unit. He's shouting but it's so hard to hear in the full PPE, and through masks, and over alarms, in this high-ceilinged echo warehouse. As we talk, and he updates me on the state of the patients, I watch a nurse a few feet away caring for a patient who is lying face down, hooked up and attached, almost bionic and robotic, half-human, half-machine. There is no detail of her patient to give her clues about her life, but I learn she is fifty years old. The nurse, too, looks around the same age. Midlife women, like me. The nurse is performing tasks that I know and understand, but this is a new disease, a new and unknown environment, and everything is so much harder with the space suits. The patient is unconscious, paralysed and sedated as all the patients, in a medical coma in order to tolerate the artificial ventilation. The numbers on her monitor are not stable, and I can see, even in the short time I stand here, that things are getting worse despite maximum support from the ventilator. The nurse is rushing around. But she stops at the end of her bed. I can see that she is crying, broken. I do not know the patient, or the nurse, these two women on the opposite sides of this fence, thrown together unexpectedly. We do not have enough nurses. The shortage of critical care nurses is one of the most significant challenges: we have poached nurses and doctors from all corners imaginable for this makeshift place. We have school nurses, orthopaediac consultants, dentists, even cabin crew, all trying to figure out the job of a critical care nurse, an impossible ask. I am in awe of these colleagues, this pick-and-mix team of people walking towards danger to help others, strangers, some who might deserve help, and some who might not, regardless. Reminding me what is important in life. This is a time of dehumanisation. And yet in many ways, this feels like the most human time of all. I love and am loved, and it all, here, becomes clear, that life is a blessing.

And in this place, right here and now, my reaction to my perimenopause feels utterly farcical. My quest for romantic love, obsessing over my body, clear fear of ageing, have been a waste of precious time, of this precious, precarious life. This critical care ward full of patients with Covid is the most terrifying place I've ever seen. But this room also contains the only things that matter, or should matter, to all of us. This hospital, like all hospitals and healthcare settings around the entire world at this moment in history, is full of terror. But it is also full of love, compassion, kindness, empathy and grace. These people, both patients and staff, contain all the meaning in the universe, the reason we are here: for each other.

What a privilege to be here, midlife, and have the chance to change.

The nurse looks up at her patient, and along the row of other patients, and then she looks at the ceiling of this cold, lifeless place. And she bends her head, puts her hands together in front of her chest. I wonder if she is religious. Or atheist. Or if that even matters at all. At this time we are all praying.

The hospital walls are lined with notes and cards and messages.

To the doctors and nurses looking after our mum, thank you. We love our mum, and we love you too.

We can't put into words what you have done for us. Unreal. Thank you.

You are in our thoughts and prayers, along with our grand-dad. Stay strong.

We know you are doing all you can for my husband. Be safe.

We thank you at this terrible time, for doing your best for us all.

From our family. We are all one family now. Thank you.

To the staff caring for our brother, we are praying for you, too.

The team caring for my sister. We love you.

Thank you for sending the heart poem, which we received.

Thank you for the knitted heart.

These messages, from the relatives of the patients to the staff caring for their loved ones, are from strangers. And yet the very word stranger has morphed. In this dehumanising period of suffering, nobody is a stranger any more. The word 'stranger' derives from Latin, also meaning foreigner, or alien, and yet we recognise something in each other right now, a common humanity. Fear connects us. Love does. What a gift it is, to experience life and love. To have friends and family – and sometimes strangers – who really care. A nurse knits hearts, two per patient. The idea is that if a person dies, one knitted heart goes with that person, in the shroud, to the mortuary.

And the other is given to the relative. Something to hold on to. To connect. To connect the relative with the loved one they lost, but also to feel the greater connection outside that, to the person who performed this act of kindness, going the extra mile, the stranger caring for the person they love, who is not a stranger at all.

A neighbour is shielding so can't get to the shops. I offer to do some shopping for her when I do mine. She's one of those people, those older women, who I consider as having their shit together. She remembers anniversaries, is on the school governing board and facilitates the neighbourhood watch meetings. Before Covid I saw her run past my house every day, looking cheerful, as I scowled in my dressing gown. She was always disapproving of me, I felt, and of my chaos. I assumed. Within the first week of the pandemic, I am coming home from work when I see her curtains twitch, and she opens the window. 'I'm shielding, don't come near,' she shouts, but I hear the fear in her voice. 'I wonder if you might do me a favour?' The first shopping list she writes me is for eggs, smoked salmon, teabags and chicken. The next list includes red wine. By the time we're three weeks in, she texts me. 'Can you get me any weed?'

I laugh. 'Sadly no but Pete at number 257 is a smoker. Try there.'

'You must think I'm a terrible person.'

'No. I think you're human.'

We are all a bit broken. All a bit mad. Nobody has their shit together, no matter how they present to the world. And once we recognise that in ourselves, in others, really see each other, we can find connection, even love. Bernice Neugarten was an American psychologist specialising in adult, rather than child development, meaning the process of growing, changing and learning as we age. She described midlife as an experience that was necessarily traumatic. I hear a lesson of midlife, through this awful suffering. We are all human and vulnerable and messy right now, us terrible, glorious humans. The entire world seems to be searching for sudden meaning; we're consumed with it. Humanity feels to be at the top of the mountain vantage point, and we are desperate to make sense of this, our human condition, the state of us, who we are and why this has happened. Why am I here?

Maybe perimenopause is a time of reckoning? Maybe this too is a time of reckoning? The world is so polarised and divided, full of anger and hate and echo chambers and fighting and inequalities. Yet our values are shifting rapidly, almost overnight – away from the cult of youth, materialism, individualism, external beauty. None of us is a shiny version of ourselves at the moment, and we don't want to see shiny versions of others. We see strength not in the Instagram influencers out on a beach in Dubai, but in the haunted eyes of the healthcare workers. It feels like progress. An unexamined life is no longer

an option; there is no more sitting on the fence of humanity.
The concrete steady ground many felt underneath us has morphed into a black hole of uncertainty. We *all* live in the margins.
The in-between, the space in the centre of the before, and the
after. And we don't really seem to understand what it's for, but
we all feel this sea change, of society, and culture, and humanity
itself. The transformation happening externally but inwardly
too. We are changing.

'You can come out now,' I repeat, as I step out of the bathroom,
wet and wrapped in a dressing gown.

They run at me, almost knocking me over, these teens who
are taller than I am already, yet still so, so young. My children
who drive me mad with frustration and make me angry and
exhausted and exasperated and guilty and unhinged. They
lean into me, and breathe, as though they've been holding their
breath for a long time, and I smell them, and breathe them in
too, touch the warmth of their skin, put a hand on their chests,
feeling each of their heartbeats, both strong, fast, sure. Then I
put my arms around them both, their heads on my shoulders,
and we stay motionless, eyes closed, and this single moment
feels like forever.

We hug each other, tighter than we have ever hugged
before.

9

A Car Park, in the Rain: Love

Pre-Covid. The worst holiday. Joy and I both need a holiday, we're exhausted by life, but we're also skint. She has talked me into booking the cheapest cruise on the internet. 'I'll book it on credit card, you can pay me back in instalments.'

I have never, ever, wanted to go on a cruise. 'It's for ancient people,' I say. 'Rich, old folk.'

But Joy has this idea in her head, fuelled by a notion of something that, I suspect, doesn't exist any more, one of old-fashioned politeness and proper glamour. At least, it doesn't exist on the type of cruise we are booking. I look at the price. 'That seems suspiciously cheap for even a cheap cruise.'

'It's fifty pounds a person cheaper to have no window,' she tells me, and for some reason, I neither question this nor visualise a submarine. We're going through the mill, exhausted and full of responsibilities, and she's organised childcare for both of us, and her enthusiasm is infectious. 'The high seas,' she says, 'dressing for dinner. An escape from our lives for a whole week.'

She has me at escape.

We board the boat, looking at the other passengers, who are mostly in their eighties and nineties. They look at us suspiciously. It's true we are wearing Topshop playsuits, bought in the sale, and for some unknown reason, I've shaved half my head, perhaps thinking it makes me look edgy. 'That's a terrible haircut,' Joy says. And then she covers her mouth. 'I'm going to be sick.' She looks green around the edges.

'Are you OK?'

She holds on to a barrier, and sways. 'It's just a bit choppy.' The boat is yet to move.

'I get terrible seasickness,' she continues. 'I think I'm going to throw up.' And then she lies down on the floor. Soon, a crowd gathers. Her Topshop playsuit is riding up and I start panicking that she's wearing no underwear. But I see a flash of knickers, thank God. An elderly man with a walking stick is trying to help her up. Eventually a few crew members help carry her to the dining hall, a place that, despite the brochure, smells of chlorine and looks like a hospital canteen. This ship is not high end. Joy is seasick. We have yet to leave the dock. I'm wondering whether to just get straight off. Joy is lying on the floor, with her hands dramatically over her head. A waiter arrives with a tray, gestures to the canteen area. 'Can I get you some food? It might settle your stomach?'

He looks at me and I see in his face that he's used to dealing with drama.

Joy lowers her hand. 'Maybe chicken,' she says.

I kneel next to her and whisper, 'Get up, you're really embarrassing.' I've known her long enough to know when she's over-dramatising for attention. She loves attention. There is no possibility of Joy sinking into the background at midlife, becoming invisible. She's like a flaming comet, gaining heat with every minute. 'Not that bit,' she waves her hand towards the waiter picking out a piece of chicken from a nearby tray. 'The plumper one at the back.'

Joy has always been larger than life, dramatic, unashamed, filling up every room she goes into with laughter and light. I love her confidence. Like all my friends, she's not one thing or another, but she's all the things. She's a great mum, a brilliant nurse, a loyal friend, and she's a proudly difficult woman with little to no shame. I love being around her, as someone who feels ashamed most of the time. She is fearless. She doesn't care what other people think. A skill I am yet to learn, but perhaps that I'm finally edging towards.

After a few days on the awful boat, Joy recovers and is back to her full self. She signs herself up for the talent show, and I dread to ask her what the talent will be. She has the worst singing voice of any person I've ever heard and she loves singing and refuses to do it quietly. But it's worse than that. I look at the list on the bar door:

Joy: Burlesque.

I have never wanted the ground to swallow me up so much as watching Joy dance on that cruise. Watching the people watching her. Elderly people, mostly. One man, I notice, has an oxygen mask. I scan the area for a defibrillator. A woman who looks around our age, yet is dressed and behaving like someone our age, wearing something other than Topshop, and certainly not dancing in the manner we do, tuts repeatedly, and I think of my great nan, and bitter disappointment.

After the performance we leave the shell-shocked guests and return to our windowless cabin. Joy puts on some music and we talk and talk. We talk about our messy lives, we laugh hysterically above the bass. After a few hours, a loud thud on the door.

The disapproving woman from earlier is standing there, with her hair in rollers, wearing a dressing gown, or at least, I think it's a dressing gown. It looks more like a housecoat that my nan might wear while baking. I want to ask about the rollers and why she'd bring a dressing gown on a cruise, but I don't have time. She's shouting. Joy turns the music down.

'You two, how old are you? You're behaving like teenagers.

It is three o'clock in the morning, and I can hear your music, and I can hear every word you two are saying. And I mean every single word.'

I apologise and scan backwards through our conversations. I feel bad that we've been so inconsiderate, disrespectful and frankly annoying. But Joy just turns on the music again. And she says, 'we might be behaving like teenagers but who writes those rules anyway? We'll never be as young as we are today. And we're planning to enjoy it.'

Shortly after this holiday, Joy gets a cancer diagnosis. And I'm so glad we went on that awful cruise; and more than that, it turns out it wasn't awful at all, but the best of times. I'm glad Joy and I spent all night laughing and talking. And I'm even glad she did her burlesque in the crappy cruise talent contest.

I can't believe I didn't win!'

You were robbed!

In *At The Existentialist Café*, philosopher Sarah Bakewell describes her student experience as transformative: 'I managed to spend my days and evenings more or less as the existentialists had in their cafés: reading, writing, drinking, falling in and out of love, making friends, and talking about ideas. I loved everything about it, and thought that life would always be one big existentialist café.' Of course, life is not one big existentialist café, and is full of regrets but I never ever regret having fun with my friends. We can be debauched, temporarily irresponsible, wild and silly. I wish I'd done more of it.

Joy and her husband Sebastian are the people I write down in my will, the night before I return to Covid ICU, who I would like to care for my children. I think about that a lot. Joy's wildness, her eccentricities and the loudness of her. Her courage. How she really is her name. And I can't think of anyone in the world who would care for and love my children as much as I do. I'd trust her with my life. I think about that woman knocking on our door at 3 a.m. How much she judged us, especially Joy. How I judged the woman too. How little she saw, or understood, from the outside. How little I did. I wonder how little we all understand of each other, from the outside.

I'd give anything to go back. But at least, like Joy said, we've broken open. We can see inside each other a bit more clearly. The bad, as well as the good. I'd give anything to go back and be on that awful boat with my friend. I'd invite the woman knocking on our door at 3 a.m. into our horrible cabin. She looked like she could use some friends. I am so lucky, to have such friends in my life. To be surrounded with love. To be surrounded with friends who truly believe that age is just a number, those who understand there are many ways to be a woman.

Mirren is drinking hot chocolate from a flask in the park. People walk past huddled against the cold, turning their heads to look at her. She is my most glamorous friend. I have never seen her without perfect make-up and hair, immaculate manicured nails. Not even now, mid-lockdown. 'I watched YouTube videos,' she says. She's beautiful and sexy too. And she happens to be seventy. 'What's your upper age range? I'll set you up.'

She notices my pursed lips, frown, and rolling eyes. Despite being a dear friend and wanting the best for me, last time she set me up was with a man who I had literally nothing in common with. She is single, and has a lifetime of love stories, yet despite the traumas she carries, believes in love. Wants it for me. She is such a generous and warm soul. When she gets a cat from Battersea, she says she is done with dating, but still, wants a 'beating heart next to hers'.

'I'm through with dating. Seriously.'

'Look,' she carries on. 'How bad can it be? We're in a pandemic.'

But of course, with each fling, each relationship, each bad one – there is trauma, and a risk that you bring that into the next relationship. The chance of happiness becomes less and less sure, as new hurts chip away. To continue to search for love at midlife and beyond takes an optimism that is at once brave and stupid. A risky business. We discuss this and many other things too. I look to her for wisdom about love. Despite refusing her offer of a set-up. She has seen it all and got the T-shirt and made sense of it and peace with it.

'I'm honestly done finding love. I'm finished with dating. I don't want, or need a partner or spouse. In fact, searching for one has done me more harm than good.'

'You don't need a forever partner to live a fulfilled life,' she agrees. 'Some rare people are lucky to have that. But you do need love stories.'

She's so wise, Mirren. She is another of the older women I admire who I am gradually surrounding myself with. I am lucky enough to have many of them in my life: these older, wild, glamorous, sexy, incredibly visible women who remind me what might be possible as I age. Women who are a bit rough around the edges, who know stuff. I remember as a young girl scouring beaches for the prettiest shells, delighting as I found the smooth, shiny, perfect ones, and putting them in my bucket. Now I am collecting once more, though the heavy pebbles with rough edges feel like the real treasure. Archaeologist Rebecca Wragg Sykes describes the prettiness of flint, how easy it is to dig for analysis, as opposed to silcretes, which she spends three years researching nonetheless. I learn from her that you need to dig really deep for silcretes, a hard and resistant material used to make tools. She tells me that it is often seen as undateable, unattractive, redundant, and it was never straightforward to find, but it is worth the search: *we discovered incredible colours in re-silification: pinks, blues, oranges and reds.*

'I no longer want or care about a sandy beach. Just the sea,' I say.

Mirren laughs. 'You talk a lot of shit.'

We both laugh. It's true, I do. Mirren drinks her hot chocolate, and we watch the park, taking deep breaths of cold air. 'What a time.'

We talk about our respective families, our struggles, work stress, financial worries, the weight of womanhood. And we talk about what might happen to the world, speculate about the state of the economy, the collective depression that seems to have covered the country, the world.

'It's as if the whole world has aged overnight,' she says. 'We have psychological arthritis. Inevitable, incurable pain.'

A giant black dog runs past us. We both look at the dog, each other, then laugh. 'Case and point,' she says.

'Wasn't it Stephen Hawking who said, life would be tragic if it wasn't so funny?'

She nods. 'We're in the "life would be funny if it wasn't so tragic" phase. We're all just doing our best to get through the day. One moment at a time.'

I think about Orla, who phoned me earlier, and how she is struggling, too. 'My entire list. Everything on the Fuck It Bucket List gone up now in a puff of smoke. I mean what am I to write on it now? Bake some bread? It's hardly going to be soul-enhancing. There isn't any yeast anywhere anyway.'

And she's right, nothing feels soul-enhancing right now. Everything seems to be coated with a layer of drizzle, a mist of apathy. We are all anxious, and a bit depressed, in a shared mood that gains collective power. Of course, Covid is a storm in which we find ourselves in different boats. Orla and I discuss climate change, the existential threats to democracy, racism, gender-based violence, poverty and loneliness, and the mental health crisis that is coming over the horizon like a tsunami. But amidst this discussion her Fuck It Bucket List doesn't lose any potency; if anything it gains it. More than ever we need to remember to live, and consciously carve out the life we want, if we possibly can. The illusion of control has disappeared, and it is clear to all of us that the control we thought we had over our lives was not ours at all. We are all blowing around in the wind, imagining we are dancing.

Saturday begins as normal. I get up, make coffee and shout at my daughter to get ready for dance. She attends an advanced dance training programme and has not missed dance lessons of any kind since she was a toddler. She danced her way through missed birthday parties and holidays, through swine flu and post-surgery. Yet today, she says she's not well. I poke my head in. Her bedroom is painted dark purple, almost black, the walls covered with photographs of her and friends pulling stupid faces, and the surfaces with Mexican Day of the Dead memorabilia. She's never been to Mexico. On the floor lie piles of clothes that we argue about continuously (Clean? Dirty? Textiles homework?) I count six cups on her desk as well as a mouldy banana skin, a bowl containing a foul-smelling concoction made from rice water that she learnt from a YouTube clip is good for her hair, and a dog lead. We do not own a dog. I'm about to complain about the clothes, banana peel, cups, foul-smelling rice-water hair mask, and ask about the dog lead, but notice she has her eyes closed. Usually when I go into her room she glares at me in horror, as if I'm walking on sacred ground rather than dirty (or clean or textiles homework) clothes. She hisses at me to Wait For A Reply After Knocking Do You Not Understand Privacy, but today she doesn't say a word. She's so hot I can feel her temperature before my hand touches her forehead. I take a few moments outside her bedroom and feel the weight of my choices press onto my body, the back of my head, my teeth. I've been working as a nurse in a Covid hospital through this first peak; her dad and his partner are also doctors on the frontline. We are a high-risk family. I have come home after twelve or more hours, scrubbed my clothes, keys, body, phone, hair, thrown everything into a hot wash and only then told the kids they can come out of their rooms. But being meticulous hasn't been enough. I try not to let that sink in yet. I shout for my son to stay in his room, open all the windows and shut my daughter's before disappearing downstairs to get paracetamol and water and a thermometer to give my nurse-heart a number it already knows: 40. By noon she can't stand. And by nightfall we are in Main Resus at King's College Hospital, and she is on the edge of life.

There is nothing in the world more frightening than understanding that your child might die. Nothing. That knowledge contains all the darkness of the universe. At first, I refuse to acknowledge even the flicker of the thought. A junior doctor takes me aside as they do bloods, and begin fluid resuscitating her, pushing in bags of saline, and she is semi-conscious, drifting in and out of herself, of this world. 'It's pretty serious,' he says. 'Her blood pressure is dangerously low.' As a lifetime children's nurse I know a few things to be true. Children hold their blood pressure until the last moment. They *compensate*. The blood pressure of a child can be completely normal until moments before the end. Clever things. The physiology of childhood is fascinating. 'A low blood pressure in a child is a medical emergency. They are decompensating, and hypotension can mean imminent cardiac arrest.' I hear my own words coming out of my mouth as I teach other healthcare professionals over the years. I hear them echo around the room, bounce off the walls, screech. I want to unknow what I know. Instead, I push away even the possibility. She will not die. That is not even imaginable on any horizon. An absolute impossibility.

I call my son every hour. I imagine his face, at home alone, pressed against the glass, looking out into the darkness. The worry he contains. I have no idea what to do. I can't leave my daughter. I have no family within a hundred miles. She likely has Covid, meaning he might, and needs to isolate. Yet he is alone, and I am here. My head is scrambled egg. Much of single parenting is crisis management, trying to solve impossible practical puzzles. I can't leave him all night. I can't leave her. It's a choice between bad and worse, not good and better solutions. I do what I always do in moments of need. I call Joy, wake her up.

I mumble a few words, my voice scratchy and breaking. She doesn't need to hear the details. Our language of friendship means she can hear pain and the extent of it, without words. 'I'll get in the car now,' she says. 'I'll keep him until whenever. Don't worry about him. Focus on her.'

I breathe. Good friends help you breathe. Joy has her own stresses. She is working full time as a nurse, and mum to three sons. 'We're family,' she says, as if reading my thoughts.

'He might have Covid. I don't want to put you at risk. Put the boys or Sebastian at risk. I can't. But I don't know what to do.'

'There's only one solution here. We'll take him and all isolate. And if we get it, we get it. He's your son so he's my son too.'

This is the early days of Covid. Before tests are freely available. We none of us know how it will affect us. Whether if we catch it, we'll get sick, or even die. Joy is quite literally risking her health, and her life, to save mine. Unconditional love is not only reserved for lovers and children, it can happen in friendships too.

After an Emergency Department night, of pacing the hallways, and thinking of all the parents over the years I cared for, who paced the hallways too, she is well enough to be transferred to a ward. We end up on the oncology ward, now turned Covid ward. 'Stay in the room,' a nurse tells us, through thick PPE. Every few minutes during the night she comes in, quietly, and checks the drip, gives medication, takes observations. I watch her breathing, protective, suspicious, and totally filled with dread. 'Her blood pressure is still low,' I say. 'It doesn't seem to be picking up with fluid.'

I think of inotropes, the strong heart medications that can help with blood pressure in the critically ill. Those drugs you can only receive on intensive care. And I know they are wondering about that. The intensive care consultants, who I know very well, pop over during the night, to say hello, in their bright and breezy voices.

'Are you causing problems, sweetheart? Just like your dad!' And they smile at me with their eyes and give me illegal hugs. But I watch their eyes skim over her blood pressure, and a glimmer of something I understand. I wish I didn't.

PIMS-TS is something that most people have never heard of, and I have never really heard of, until this time. 'We're seeing loads of kids with this,' a nurse tells me. 'Mainly black and mixed-race teens for some reason. Really low blood pressure. They're in intensive care on inotopes sitting up and talking. It's really weird.'

For two days everyone thinks this is what is wrong with my daughter. That she has a rare, post-viral version of Covid. I begin to hear stories from nurse friends who are caring for these children. Some are developing heart problems, cardiomyopathy, and a few are having strokes. It's hard to even contain that information in my head. She gets slightly worse. A C Reactive Protein, or CRP, is a measurement that indicates how unwell a person is. In a sick person, a CRP might rise to 10. In the very sick, 100. Some of the sickest children I have ever looked after had CRPs of 200. Children who have tragically died.

Her CRP is 300.

She has echo after echo, heart scans done by the most senior specialists, and I sit in the dark room watching her insides, hearing the whoosh, watching the eyes of the consultants performing the scans. I watch the colours inside her, the structures she's made of, the possibilities contained in all of us that can change in a heartbeat. They can't see any changes. 'Yet,' one of them says to me.

And every conversation and piece of information I do not want to hear is contained in that single word.

A nurse comes in, to do observations and check on us. 'So you worked in Covid ICU,' she says, 'and dad is an intensivist?'

I nod, watch my daughter, who is far away and somewhere else.

The nurse squeezes my shoulder. 'I can't imagine.'

And I can't imagine. Even now. But the thought keeps infiltrating all others: *She might die. You gave her this virus, and now she might die.*

But she doesn't die. A few more unstable days and they eventually find a bacterial infection in her urine, a problem on the kidney scan. 'It looks like sepsis. Urosepsis.'

And sepsis is a nightmare. I have cared for so many children with sepsis, too many who did not make it. They swarm around my head like bees, images I wish I could be rid of. They change IV antibiotics, and give more fluid, and clotting factors, and gear up for intensive care, but just like that she turns a corner.

I hear myself in so many interviews talking about why I chose children's intensive care as a nursing career. I hear my own voice talking to Luisa.

Children get very sick very quickly. But with the right staff, and the right technology, they can get better very quickly too.

I have never, ever felt more grateful to live in a country where healthcare is treated as a human right, regardless. Where the skill and expertise of the best nurses and doctors in the world have literally saved my daughter's life. I have never been so grateful to live in a time when we have the technology that can help people survive even sepsis. We are lucky. Today, we are lucky.

I think about gratitude. Privilege. I am overwhelmed with feeling so incredibly grateful. Perspective is a funny thing. The agonising year I've spent searching for a way out of melancholy, and sadness, and hopelessness, and yet in the midst of death and disease and loss, the time of Covid shakes me alive again.

I think of all the things I worry and obsess about, those things that can seem so incredibly important. As she sleeps, I google the name I gave her that seemed so important and true and a gift for her: Bella – *beautiful*. I go over the conversations we've had about her wanting a new name, how she has been flirting with identity, exactly as she should be as a teen, trying out and finding out who she is becoming. Rowan – meaning a tree of life that symbolises courage, wisdom and protection. I discover that rowan trees can grow in the most difficult of places, even in thin, acid soil, and are frost-hardy and wind-resistant with the deepest of roots.

'Rowan,' I whisper. And she opens her eyes.

'Can we get a dog?' She sits up slightly for the first time in a week. She is skeletal, skinny before and with no reserves. Her eyes are shadowed dark, and I can see her heart working so hard, pulsating in her neck.

Life is a heartbeat.

'We can get a dog,' I say. Frankly, I'd get her a giraffe. 'Yes. We can get a dog.'

Covid, like the perimenopause, has stripped me bare, made me feel as if I've lost my entire identity. The trauma of living through an internal as well as external change has forced to the surface all my anxieties and vulnerabilities. The physical expressions of insomnia, anxiety, hair loss, have increased: my body is still trying to speak what my conscious mind is unable to process. But I now believe in fate, in a way that I did not before. The random nature of life with no pattern is a pattern in itself. There's no control. At least, not in the way I'd imagined. Simply chaos. But for me at least, there is accept-ance in that understanding. I'd always felt a bit out of control, and chaotic, in a way I imagined others weren't. Other women seemed to project calm, organised togetherness. Now we're all chaos. And I realise we probably always were. Nothing is cer-tain, nor has it ever been. The loss of that realisation is frightening, but it's freeing too. We're standing on quicksand. We always were.

There are many lessons from this time, but perhaps the most urgent is the lesson I keep going back to, the one that my dad was trying to tell me.

Love each other. Love is the only thing that matters, in the end.

I have held on too tightly to my dad's words, until they became squeezed and misshapen, distorted. I don't think he was talking about romantic love, not at all. During this time that I consciously decide not to try and find love, I realise I am surrounded by it. I begin to take walks. I've always loved walking, but the mega walks get longer and longer, and my mind empties for the first time in months. I can breathe. I am completely in the present moment, able to put one foot in front of the other, to look at the trees at dusk and marvel at the stars. After being up close and personal to suffering, it feels like a miracle that I get this chance to simply live, and I am grateful. Nothing is perfect. Maybe it never will be. But I don't need to wait for perfect to be happy. Happy can happen in the sticky margins of life. Love is everywhere. Even in this. Especially in this.

I realise that we are all living in a time when it is impossible to tell where one human being ends and another begins.

We are so interconnected. It's frightening. But if we lean into it, the idea that we are all, each and every one of us, despair and hope and terror and beauty, that we are vulnerable and broken and completely and totally interconnected, we find that we are love itself. I have been searching and searching for love stories in all the wrong places, but they were there all along. I'm surrounded by love. And the love stories of my life are my children, family and friends, and my work, and now, after this time of intense change, I'm even learning to love myself, a bit. Midlife, and Covid, are times for so many of us of profound suffering. But they are also ones of profound love. As well as love stories, I realise. I'm learning about acceptance and gratitude and hope. We are blowing around in the wind, it is true, but sometimes, we're also dancing.

Ben contacts me on social media: he's doing a series of talks about compassion, and has come across my first memoir about nursing, *The Language of Kindness*. He sends a nice, though to be fair, very long message, about how we knew each other at school, we were friends, and he was also a friend of my brother, and my mum taught us both at nursery school, where we went together aged three, and we were born in the same hospital – do I remember him? And at first, I have no clue. My longer-term memory is not good, and I have clearly not stayed in touch with him over the years. I ran as fast as I could away from Stevenage, away from home.

But then I remember.

Ben, who was wise, even when we were teens.

Bible Ben!

Of course I remember. I think back to the bins, after my first-ever dating experience, where Arron did not show up and I was heartbroken. *He doesn't deserve you.* I did not believe

Ben then, and of course, I remain undeserving, but Ben has devoted his life to others. He tells me about the food bank he's been running for six years, the difficulties during Covid of keeping it going, despite a huge increase in demand. I can't imagine how impossible it has been, how hard he is working. He has swallowed all the goodness of the world.

'We could have coffee and a walk,' he tells me. 'Be lovely to catch up properly. How long has it been since we last saw one another? Thirty years? Wow – we've known each other for forty-one years.'

And we work out that outside my family he's the person who I've known longest in the world.

I have no idea if he's suggesting coffee as an actual date, or even if he's flirting full-stop. As such old friends it's natural and familiar when we chat, and I wonder if I'm reading into it. But we message anyway, become friends again. We are middle-aged now, and our lives are so complex and have been full of suffering as well as joy. A life without such texture and complexity is simply going through the motions. Not really living. I always wanted to live with my eyes wide open. Nursing allowed me to do that. Midlife is allowing that too. Even the pandemic has meant that my vision is sharp and I can't look away. All the sadness is filling me up and yet I am not empty, not even in my biggest spaces, or darkest gaps. For I am full of the precious nature of humanity. Ben and I have huge responsibilities and there's a whole heap of people relying on us both, and we have completely different lives in many ways. Our lives have transformed into something multi-layered and much more abstract, more challenging. Change is the work. I think of all my previous selves, contained inside me, slightly different, smaller versions of who I am, like a Russian Doll. I'm still all those people, but I've got extras now too. And layers that are well hidden from most people. But not from Ben.

We arrange to meet at Regent's Park, and I see him outside the tube. We are both older. But somehow, he looks the same. And although we are grown-ups, within seconds of talking, I see that we're both still really those awkward teenagers, rebellious in opposite ways: me with a badge that says, Fuck Off, Ben, quietly reading. It's as if no time has passed at all, and we're standing outside the bins, and fourteen years old instead of forty-something. I look at him and my body knows him. It's like muscle memory or alchemy. He's at once familiar and new. We have so much to catch up on, so many years and gaps, and yet walking around the park it's as if we have spent the last thirty years walking around the park.

I collect Ben things in my head, the way I tease his big ears, how his skin can be hot in one area and cold in another, his endless kindness, his enthusiasm for chilli seeds and coupons. He always has change and carries stamps, which cracks me up. We are the total opposite and the total same.

I hear Luisa's voice in my head. *Love isn't a quilt on fire, that's just an activated attachment pattern.*

There is nothing on fire about Ben. Nothing dangerous. He offers to take my nan a food parcel. He buys me a jar of cheap coffee. (*I know you love NHS coffee. Keep going with writing. I am with you.*) He offers to pop over one lunchtime – he has made dinner for me and the kids to *save me cooking later*. He drops off dinner on the doorstep, then leaves. It's a five-hour round trip. He is steady. Calm. Present. Honest. It is wildly unnerving. When he asks me out, on a proper date, a more-than-friends date, my instinct is to run. I'm about to put a stop to our chatting, and explain that I am not in a place where I'm interested in love, or even believe in dating, and then I hear Luisa's voice in my head, again, loud and clear, almost shouting:

Giant Dolphin. Huge gigantic fucking dolphin.

Not that Luisa would swear. But these are the words in my head.

I have been on hundreds of dates in my life. But the best date of my life happens with my friend Ben, during a pandemic, when we go to Morrisons, buy some cheap breaded ham and bread, and eat it on the car park wall, in the rain.

We sit on a cold wall and talk and talk and talk. Everything he says feels measured and important. He always was wise. Time seems to gallop as we sit here, and one hour turns into four. My hair is wet, but despite my pathological fear of the cold, I am warm. He asks if he might kiss me. I have kissed so many people. A lot of frogs. And I've had some amazing kisses too. But kissing Ben is something close to spiritual. He tastes of orange Fanta. And we are briefly and totally connected to each other in a profound way.

We are both quiet a while after kissing, unable to speak. Then we laugh. I watch the electric air, the drizzle, the now endlessly beautiful car park. Ben puts his arm around me, and we huddle together and talk more, listen more, absorb more. The light is changing. The car park is emptying slowly of shoppers. If I could pause the world in this moment, I would, and stay here forever.

Ben sighs. He touches my cheek with his fingertips, and looks at me as I've never been looked at before. Like he sees right though my skin to my insides. 'Well,' he says.

'Well then,' I say. And we laugh.

10

Leaping Towards
the Sky: Change

The only day in my life so far where I feel I have it together,
and I'm a sophisticated and possibly even glamorous, mature
woman. There's a glitzy award ceremony in central London,
and I have spent a week preparing: hair masks, face masks,
moisturising my entire body to within an inch of my life, planning an outfit, nails. Choosing a dress takes many weeks. It has
to be perfect. I feel great. The day finally arrives and I've forgotten to take the bins out – but nothing will stress me – I'll
simply drop off the rubbish at the tip en route to the awards.
We have a big problem with foxes (I later find out my neighbour has been leaving eggs out to feed them, and occasionally
offal) and awards or not, the bins are only collected every two
weeks. I've arranged childcare and give myself plenty of time
for a detour. There is no way I'll be late. Everything is organised, and running to plan. I remember feeling very pleased
with myself. I'm not yet perimenopausal but I have a sense that
I'll age well, become more not less, grow not shrink into a

civilised and suave woman: I'll sail through the next half of my life in a Chanel Number 5 mist of high class. My heels are high, but even these I can walk in, as though it is effortless. I think of the speech, holding the award in my hand, how many famous people I'll get to schmooze with, and the champagne I'll drink. As a newly sophisticated woman, I'll drink with far more decorum than in the past, when a free bar to me meant I had to drink all of it. Now, I will sip a glass, and have a canapé and everything will be measured, and controlled and moderate. I will no longer be a young woman of extremes and chaos, but a fully-fledged grown-up.

The smell from Bromley refuse centre does not cut through the amount of perfume I've sprayed on. I put a long coat over my evening dress – a sequin gown that has cost me a fortune. I've spent a month dress shopping. I've worked so hard for so many years; I want to mark the occasion properly. Any smells from the tip will not land on the dress, as my coat is wound tightly around me. I carry the rubbish and throw two large black sacks into the skip 'general household waste'.

As soon as I've done it, I realise.

My car key has flown in, with the rubbish. I look around for someone to help, but everyone in a hi-vis jacket is far away, and looks busy. The skip is nearly full; I can probably reach it. Nothing will rain on my parade today.

I reach, and reach, and stretch as far as I can, and it is just out of my grasp, but the high heels give me extra length and so I manage to grab. I feel the edge of the car key in my hand, and I'm about get hold of it. And then I fall. I land on a dirty, stained mattress, between the bags of rotting rubbish, and my Chanel Number 5 is immediately replaced with the smell of haddock. I hear my nan's wise voice in my head: *pride always comes before a fall.* The refuse collectors are suddenly here, in front of the skip, laughing. I look down. My coat has come undone.

'Need a hand, love,' they say.

I do not like being laughed at. But my sophisticated non-chalance has left me. And instead of feeling like I have my shit together at last, and I'm the kind of woman I admire and want to emulate, I realise I am as messy and silly and immature as I ever had been. I am simply a woman in a sequin dress in a skip.

Growing up has not correlated at all with growing older. In my teens I assumed that at eighteen I would magically, and mysti-cally, somehow be an adult. It is still yet to happen. Moving through my forties has not been what I thought it would. The physical shock of perimenopausal symptoms nearly sent me spiralling out of control. Even with HRT, which in my case helped me, there was so much to process and unpick. Ageing has not come gently, or quietly. There is no elegantly slipping towards enlightenment and wisdom. It's been more of a process of undiscovery than discovery, a disentangling of my perceived self, a painful digging to get at my core. I spent a lifetime searching: for meaning, love, faith even, and yet it has all been outward looking. At midlife I begin a new journey inwards. Midlife brings its own meaning, layers of richness, to the very heart of me – the identity inside my deep insides. All along, it turns out, I've been looking for myself. Seemingly overnight, I realise that the self I thought I knew was a hologram. An imagined person. A projection. I was a knot of illusion, I had created an idea in my head of who I was, and who I was becoming, that perhaps never existed. And I have learnt that I can never be a person that I'm not, despite how hard I try. Growing older is about becoming comfortable with the person that I am, not an imaginary, wished-for version of myself. I'll *always* be a woman in a sequin dress in a skip. I am coming to realise that. American shame researcher Brené Brown reminds me in *The Gifts of Imperfection*: 'Let go of who you think you're supposed to be; embrace who you are'. I am not one thing or another. I still often feel messy and loud and disaster-prone, but I'm learning to embrace all of that. Even the chaos. In an article for *The Nation*, Toni Morrison said: 'Like failure, chaos contains information that can lead to knowledge – even wisdom.' Although I still don't feel wise, I'm at least now wise enough to surround myself with people who are. People who remind me that the threads of life are made up of light and dark and in-between spaces. I am good and bad, sensible and not. I am a grown-up, and yet full of complexity and sometimes, often, confusion. I am a mum, and daughter and sister and aunt and granddaughter and I'm a professor and nurse and writer. I'm also a teenage tearaway, a misfit, a bit awkward, full of pain and trauma as well as love and light and laughter. I am the sum of all my parts. I have swallowed suffering and love and hope. I imagine my bones, rings inside rings like the trunk of a tree. I feel vulnerable – yet stronger, too. That might be the therapy, or it might be the HRT, or it might be a swoop into gratitude, into selfhood, a combination of all these things. But whatever has helped me, that feeling of being outside my own body has disappeared, as though I've climbed back into my own skin once more. This year has been one of such intense change. The perimenopause might last up to ten years, but for me this year has been the flipping of a coin. I am not young any more. I am not old yet. I am at the perfect in-between, in the margins, the spaces and gaps. Everything is possible. I feel no fear about this change. Intrigue, and even a little excitement. I've stopped trying to be perfect. I will never be perfect.

Imperfect is beautiful. I feel like I've found the self-reflective tools Susie Orbach describes in an article for *Red* as essential in understanding life better: 'You experience something like a break-up or cancer, and that bounces you into trying to understand that life isn't black and white; it's technicolour, with all the dark colours there as well.'

Physicists are divided about the possibility of universes outside our own. Unproveable scientific theories in quantum mechanics are controversial; many are scorned, but there are some experts who believe in the theory of the *quilted multiverse*. That is, a group of multiple universes – or parallel universes – quilted together, which contain everything that exists: the entirety of space, time, matter, information and energy. Of course, there are many scientists who think the notion of multiverses a laughable pseudo-science, but central to its theory is poetry: that this, all of it, stretches on for infinity, and we continue forever. I am still searching for meaning, and I may not be finding answers, but I am finding comfort in the questions. I like theoretical physics, which seems to me at once factual and also mysterious, paradoxical in the best sense. Faith and quantum physics have things in common, I discover. Both are centrally concerned with the idea that there is more reality beyond the extent to which we can see. We are the fabric of space. My life is a patchwork quilt, a universe of galaxies and stars inside me, and it's all the more beautiful because of the colours.

I remember giving talks along with other writers to hundreds of school children in rural Nigeria as part of a festival promoting literacy. At the end of the talks, we ask the audiences: Why do you read? Why are books important? Most of the answers that come back are as expected. A few tall, older boys stand up, and explain that reading will improve their chances of gaining entry to medical/law/engineering school. But another writer tells us, over dinner, about the school she visited, and a small girl standing up – a wisp of a thing, all knees and elbows. 'I'll always remember what that little girl said, how brave she was, how clear. She had a voice so quiet that a microphone had to be found and passed to her. "I read," she said, "because I want to be a wise woman. I want to fly in colour."'

Looking back from the vantage point of midlife I can imagine giving my younger self advice. *Worry less about anything external. None of it matters.* I can also see into the future, and perhaps hear exactly the same advice from my older self. But of course, I still worry about external issues. I stare in the mirror and wonder who I am, my insides feeling stuck in teenage or twenties, and my face an older woman's. Perhaps I will always feel that way internally, baffled by my changing reflection? My nan says she feels eighteen, despite being in her nineties, and gets a shock every time she looks in the mirror. I find strange comfort in discovering I am not alone in that. I'm still preoccupied with practical and physical things too, despite developing a shift in priorities. But the questions that plagued my twenties and thirties, took so much energy and time, no longer preoccupy me: Am I good enough? Fit enough? Kind enough?

Am I working hard enough? I can be in this day, in this moment, still. This time of perimenopause feels like an opportunity, this pause, perhaps a reckoning, a crossroads: either become smaller, less visible, or perhaps grow, and demand to be seen and heard. Many of my friends are at the same stage of life, and many are older too. Grandmothers.

We are bombarded with mothers drinking gin, the 'bad moms', and the yummy-mummy school-gate-competitive narrative. But what about the grandmothers? My view and understanding of grandmothers and elderly women is changing along with my view of parenting. My perception – perhaps everyone's perception – of grandmothers or at least grandmother-aged women, is of grey-haired little ladies who store tinned food and like to knit. But of course, like everything else, this is often an illusion.

My nan always told me that when swifts arrive, summer is sure to follow. But I have another marker signalling the start of summer. It is not blossom on the trees or migrating birds or even that warm almost baked-bread smell you get in the air that tells me the season is changing. Summer always begins when I see my neighbour, Lene, who is in her seventies, in her garden eating tapas and drinking champagne with seemingly a different man every sunny evening. She is dating again. She is vibrant and energetic and kind and she's full of stories, which she bellows in a loud, unapologetic voice, laughing and laughing. I watch her from my bedroom window and smile, a woman having the time of her life, signalling summer, the ultimate in Life Goals. This is a woman who flies in colour.

When our other neighbour calls me, the reception is not great. I hear the words 'Lene married!' then the line goes dead. I try calling back, but there is no answer. I go home later, buy some flowers on the way, and pop next door to congratulate Lene and find out more. It's a sunny evening, and she's holding court in her garden, and when I walk through there are four men there. I recognise one of them who she has previously described as her dear friend who she was 'married to a million years ago'. I don't know the others. I stand awkwardly with the flowers, not quite knowing who to congratulate. I curse myself for not finding out exactly *who* Lene has married, so just say 'Congratulations' to the air and wait for one of the men to jump up. Lene throws her head back and laughs. She looks sparkling and incredibly beautiful, and I can see that she's understood my predicament and that it's also been lost on the men, who she laughingly calls later, 'gentlemen callers'. She refuses to live with her new husband, to his surprise, staying Monday to Thursday in her own place, only joining him at weekends. She tells me about her unconventional life and I watch the colour of her eyes change with the stories, from blue to green and back again. She has lived through so much. Loved and lost and loved again. 'This wine is like I am,' she tells me, sipping from her glass. 'Mature and complex, fruity with earthy notes and a romantic story or two.' She laughs and I laugh. She's a fine wine indeed. I hope to be like her one day.

Like so many of my friends, Lene is a grandmother, and full of secrets. Do all grandmothers have a cheeky, sneaky side to them?

When baby Harry is born to Joy, we are new to everything and hyper-anxious. She leaves him for the first time with her mum, who has encouraged her to take a much-needed night off, and head out for dinner. I pick her up at her mum's house as she is going through the list: organic rice cakes, bedtime routines, emergency numbers, homeopathic teething powder. Joy's mum smiles and nods and doesn't mention the four children she raised single-handedly Joy kisses Harry in his highchair, the organic rice cakes in front of him. She is crying. Separation anxiety is the real deal. When we are halfway down the road, she realises she's forgotten her purse and we head back. When we arrive, Harry has no rice cakes in front of him at all. Instead, there is a giant roly-poly and custard on his tray, in a bowl, in his hair, on his face and all over the kitchen. It smells warm and sweet and safe. I have never seen a baby look so delighted. Her mum is talking to him in a sing-song voice, having not yet noticed us return. Joy stands in horror clutching my arm. 'What she doesn't know can't hurt her,' her mum says, as Harry laughs, and grabs a handful of cake.

Another friend Corinne becomes a grandmother young, at

almost my age. Her daughter and granddaughter live with her but are staying away for the night. Corinne clears the baby equipment and monitors and takes down the kitchen gates and travel cot. She removes the fruit bowl and educational toys from the kitchen table and fills it instead with cocktail shakers and punch bowls and buckets of beers.

It's like a teenage party when the parents are away, but in reverse.

After a night of excess that ends at dawn, she replaces the fruit bowl and educational toys, and has promised to take her granddaughter to Messy Monsters, an art club for toddlers. She is wearing dark sunglasses and downing full-fat Coke. On the way home from the class, with her granddaughter in the back of the car, she becomes nauseous, despite winding down the window as far as it will go. The vomit is coming. There is nowhere to pull over safely. There is only one thing to do. She is sick into the bag containing her grandaughter's artwork. We have a long discussion about whether it's best to tell her daughter, try and clean the vomit from the art, or not mention it. Both of us agree the latter. What she doesn't know won't hurt her.

What she doesn't know won't hurt her.

How many times I have heard or said that. And yet maybe it's hurting all of us women. The more I speak, the more I share about my messy life, my disasters, pain as well as passion, the more other people share with me too. I am often humiliated, along with everyone else. Truth is a two-way mirror. In this age of perfection and projection, I am learning to live an unfiltered life. And in doing that realising that I'm not that different, or wrong or shocking than others. We're all just doing our best in this. My relationship with perfectionism is a work in progress, but I am also ambitious for other things. To be accepted and loved by people who see me exactly as I am feels like a worthy goal. I am learning new truths too. Those responsibilities I felt weighing me down at midlife are, in fact, the gifts.

I hold my children a bit tighter these days. Listen a lot more. Allow them to see me, and to know me, without hiding who I am. My imperfections. My striving. My acceptance. I enjoy taking care of my nan, being there for my mum. It feels like an enormous privilege, not a duty, to care for those around me. How lucky I am to have them around me still. I have no illusion of control these days, but I do seem to have some control over how I respond to things, how I view them. How I view myself.

Kate Bowler is a professor and author who was diagnosed with stage four cancer in her thirties. I have a conversation with her for her podcast, *Everything Happens*, that changes me. It's amazing sometimes, those people whose paths cross your own, the random conversation or the chance meeting that can have a profound effect. I have never spoken to anyone more cheerful, stubbornly hopeful or life-affirming without a hint of saccharine, who made me laugh and cry. I did not imagine I'd have much in common with this woman, a theologian and professor of the history of Christianity: our different perspectives on science and medicine seemed at odds. But as always, I am reminded how much we *all* have in common, how faith is more than religion, and sorrow and hope and love are universal. Kate has important things to say about what it means to be human, and what it means to change. She posts a blessing on social media – not something I'd subscribe to, my cynical side rolling its eyes internally, and yet I find myself nodding and nodding as I read it. She is posting, I suspect, about Covid and what we are living through. But it equally applies to perimenopause, and all the changes happening at midlife, how change is all the things:

> *Everything is different now. Your body, your age, your relationships, your job, your faith, the things that once brought you joy, the way you exist in the world. The people you love and trust and rely on.*
>
> *Things have changed. And it would be silly to imagine you haven't changed with them. You are not who you once were.*
>
> *Bless that old self. They did such a great job with what they knew.*

> *They made you who you were – all the mistakes and heartbreak and naivety and courage.*
>
> *And blessed are who you are now.*
>
> *You who aren't pretending things are the same. Who continue to grow and stretch and show up to your life as it really is. Wholehearted, vulnerable, maybe a little afraid.*
>
> *So blessed are we, The Changed.*

I am vulnerable and more than a little afraid, but I am entirely myself, the woman in a skip in a sequin dress, trying to find humour and meaning in the sticky parts of life. Instead of dread, I feel hope at the prospect of showing up to my life as it really is. That this is the beginning of change, and there will be a longer journey to examine my life, to reflect on who I am, and to let go of who I am not. I wonder if the pandemic has forced us all to take a good hard look at ourselves and work out who we are, what we want with this precious life, or if, in my case, it is perimenopause. I suspect it's a clash of both. It is not either or. Life is not in any sense binary; we hold many things at once. But whatever is creating this place of sea change, I recognise it in the eyes of all the people around me. And there is strange comfort in Kate's truth:

I am vulnerable, and a little afraid. And so are you.

We all hurt after this time, in different ways, and live with a pain that is new and hard to describe. Everyone has suffered. Yet there is a shift towards intention. The word suffer comes from *to feel keenly*. We are feeling all the feelings, and acting on them too. We lean into change. Many of my friends have decided to radically alter their lives. Teniola moves from Cheshire to Cornwall. Mirren – despite once quoting: *if it floats, fucks or flies, rent it* – sells her house and buys a houseboat. Samira comes out as non-binary. Joy and Sebastian decide to become foster parents. Sarah and her ex-husband reconcile, and embark on a polyamorous relationship. Emma begins a totally new career. Meanwhile, I have kept my promise to Rowan, and we now have a dog.

'I did not imagine that I was the sort of person who would own a Jack Russell poodle mix puppy named Gloria, yet here we are,' I tell my friends.

We are sitting on Praa Sands beach, a short drive from Teniola's new house in Cornwall. The sand is white gold in the dusk and a few surfers are trying to catch the heavy waves. We watch Gloria, the size of a cat, jumping like a kangaroo in and out of the surf. She barks at seagulls and one of them screeches back at her and she run-hops over to us, settling on Orla's lap.

'This puppy has taken over my life,' I say. 'She eats everything. Plastic, post, wires. Anything but dog food.'

'Bless her, she needs steak. Not that dry dog food. Don't you, sweet girl?' Orla scratches behind Gloria's ear. 'By the way, I've joined the Women's Institute,' she says. 'I've also started knitting.'

We all freeze, unblinking. My eyes start watering. I can feel laughter bubbling inside me, fizzing around deep down. I look around at my best friends. They are shooting burning looks at each other, lazer-eyed. Even Gloria looks up at Orla as though she does not recognise her.

Mirren breaks first. 'Fuck me, you'll be making your own fucking jam next, I expect.'

We laugh so hard I can't hear the waves. We laugh until the sky changes and a thousand stars reveal themselves. We stare at them a long time, leaning against each other, occasionally commenting on Orla's unexpected life direction. It turns out Orla has made the most radical changes to her life. Orla with her extreme bucket list of far-flung, far-out extreme adventures.

'Crochet,' she says. 'Embroidery. Zumba. Baking. I'm going to do it all. I'll even join the PTA.'

'You're not a parent or a teacher,' says Joy.

And when Orla says, 'Oh,' we laugh again.

Emma stands up and starts doing cartwheels in the sand. Teniola starts to sing. Samira lies down and makes a sand angel. Mirren is holding up a small crab to the moonlight. It's as though we are little children again. Oestrogen levels diminish post-menopause, but they don't disappear completely; I have heard that they return to pre-pubescent levels and stay there. I watch our group, imagine the other side of this, and remember exactly how it felt to be a ten-year-old girl. I think of my closeness to my grandmothers, the bond we had – still have – but particularly when I was a young girl, the shared wonder we had for the world. How Mirren is with her granddaughter, delighting in inhabiting exactly the same space, being in the moment together. I'd imagined those breathtaking, magical flashes of awe were a gift of childhood. But maybe I was wrong.

It's night now, and the sand is cold underneath us. The light has changed so quickly, and the surfers are gone. We're the only ones left on the beach. Samira sits up and puts a cardigan on. 'What's brought all this on anyway,' they ask, 'this domestic goddess new you?'

Orla gestures to the sea. 'I don't need a Fuck It Bucket List,' she says. 'I don't need it at all. It's the small things that are the big things. This right here, right now. You guys. Us. This is the adventure. We are.'

Emma stops cartwheeling and sits down. We are quiet a few moments. We look at the sky, the stars, each other, and listen to the sea, the soft howling of the wind.

'She's right,' says Mirren. And then she lowers her hand down to the sand, and watches the crab edge off it. 'Be free,' Mirren says, to the crab, or to the stars, or to us. 'Be free and live your life.'

I'm in the sea. It's not a tank after all, there is no glass. I'm surrounded by sea creatures, dangerous ones, but they are far above me and I'm in the deep blue. The bit I was most afraid of. The place in the ocean that suddenly changes colour, and I'd swim right up to it, never crossing the threshold. Now I'm in that place, far from shore. But I'm not alone here, my friends are with me. I am surrounded by them, and we're all swimming and dancing and swimming, making patterns around each other, shapes in the water. We are not alone. There are whales everywhere. Women and whales. We swim around each other, and on the seabed at the bottom of the deep blue, there is a blanket of stars. And there is glowing blue luminous plankton, and everything is magical and tiny and light. And the whales eat the plankton and we women eat the stars. And we glow in the dark.

The whole time I am dreaming about being in this giant fish tank, surrounded by sharks, I assume I am bringing the prospect of love into the therapy room. I am dreaming again. But I am in the sea, and I am with my friends, and we are swimming with whales, and I wonder if in the dream, my unconscious was processing love at all. Or if it was change.

It is the last session with Luisa. The therapy has run its course, and although she tells me that in the future I might like to have therapy again, if it is helpful, she reassures me that we've done good work to make sense of this time in my life. We talk about Ben a bit, but we don't focus on him for long.

'It seems to me,' says Luisa, smiling, 'that you're beginning to know yourself. And whatever happens with romantic relationships, Ben or otherwise, that feels like the important work.' I look at Luisa sitting underneath the window box, full of bright pink flowers. This wise woman. There is, of course, a reason we seek out help from particular people, and my subconscious pushed me towards an older woman, full of wisdom and knowledge about exactly what it means for women to age. I try to figure out if she's happy. She smiles, but not too much. Though her eyes smile too, they are also full of the sadness she has seen and been through. All of life is contained in her expression. All that she has seen and experienced and been through. All she has heard from others' lives. I wonder how many grown women, like me, she has helped to grow up. I look up at her Hokusai print. Instead of wanting to climb inside the wave and effectively drown, I notice the colours, shape and beauty of the painting. It looks nothing like I had thought. It doesn't look at all like an ending. Nor is it a beginning. It looks like the process between the two, the giant wave, a change.

'It has been described,' Luisa says, noticing me looking at the picture, 'as the sudden fury of the oceans leaping towards the sky. The artist was struck by lightning when he was fifty. Until then he had been fairly mediocre. But afterwards he did his best work.'

I play the words over and over in my head. *The sudden fury of the oceans leaping towards the sky.* I study the deep blue. I think of the recurring dream. Of the giant fish tank, and how I felt like I was inside it looking out, surrounded by my demons. I imagine my body, glowing in the dark, lit up by a thousand stars. And I realise that I am on the other side of that aquarium glass now. Perhaps perimenopause is the glass itself, not the unknown depths. The thickness of the glass depends on so many things. Culture, trauma, personality, support, society, politics. But however thin – or thick – the glass, going through it is always painful. Yet there is no way around this thing, this time, if I want to live a life whole.

'After adopting my son,' I tell her, 'I was desperate to kiss him. But he stretched his head as far from me as he could and looked away. The first six months, he would only kiss me through glass. I feel like I've been living behind glass too.' I describe my son crawling outside the living room to the other side of the glass door. Looking up at me. Leaning against the glass and pressing his face and his chubby, small hands, starfished, against the glass, making fingerprints and kiss-mark smudges, which I never cleaned. He planted his mouth against the door, and on the other side, I planted mine against his. And we did this for many, many months, protected. 'Sometimes I would try and kiss him without the glass, and he'd turn his head, eyes not finding mine. But eventually, one morning, he crawled over to me and I pulled him onto my lap, and he looked straight at me for the longest time. And he kissed me. There was nothing between us.'

'He was ready,' she says.

I am ready.

I think about the future of midlife and how that might look for women. Research into cryopreservation has already begun on the possibility of delaying menopause by twenty years. A small number of women have so far had the procedure to remove and freeze their ovarian tissue with a view to delaying the meno-pause when they are older. Doctors use keyhole surgery to remove a small piece of ovarian tissue, which is then sliced up and frozen to preserve it. When the women enter the meno-pause, potentially decades from now, the frozen tissue can be thawed out and grafted back into the body. Provided the ovar-ian tissue survives the process, it should restore the woman's declining sex hormones and halt the menopause. The proced-ure, which costs between £7,000 and £11,000, is being offered to a select number of women up to the age of forty. This process which women have always lived through, and known, and experienced, will change in the next decade or two, forever.

I think back to the first time I saw Luisa, my describing the fish finger freezer, her telling me it sounded a lot like perimeno-pause. I was so desperate then that I'd have sold all my worldly belongings for such a procedure, even after HRT patches, to avoid the suffering and symptoms I was going through, to delay getting older. But now I would always choose this, despite – or maybe because of – the forced reckoning it caused me. The shaking up of my life, my ideals, my identity.

I'm learning that pain brings something important, going through loss and change is necessary in order to experience love and hope in their most extreme forms. In an interview with *Granta*, Zadie Smith spoke of the menopause as a breakthrough: 'What a gift it is to women to have, in their own bodies, this piece of time-keeping which allows them to fully understand, in their bodies, that death is coming.'

Midlife, for me, is about crossing a threshold I never saw coming. But although I am splintered and bruised and cut from breaking through thick metaphorical glass, I can now see clearly things I did not even look at before.

'Thank you,' I say to Luisa. Of course, I am crying. I am attached to this woman who has helped me so much.

She smiles properly then, and I see a woman fulfilled.

On the way home I think of that Hokusai, and sudden fury and an ocean leaping towards the sky. I think of whales, and of women. Those mystical magical creatures full of the change, and the wonders of this universe, and this, our time. Despite the storm – or maybe because of it – the sun in the picture shines steady and high. And I realise that I am not the fisherman in the boat, clinging on for dear life. I am the wave itself, flying in colour. And I am sudden fury, leaping towards the sky.

Acknowledgements

Thank you to Sophie Lambert and the team at C&W, and Clara Farmer and the team at Chatto and Windus. To my children, for accepting that I'm not the mother of the year, and loving me anyway. And thank you to my messy, magic friends, who surround me with love, even when I am most lost. How lucky I am. This book is for you.